HOW NOT TO GET SICK WITH COLD OR FLU AND RECOVER FAST IF YOU DO

29+ Plant Based Vegan Remedies to
Strengthen Your Immune System
Which Will Help You Recover Much Faster
or Not Fall Sick With Cold or Flu at All

Ilia Zozulya

ILZ Media Publishing

ISBN 978-0-6452767-0-1 (Ebook)
ISBN 978-0-6452767-1-8 (Paperback)
ISBN 978–0–6452767–2–5 (Hardcover)

Dedication

I dedicate this book to my wife Lia.
Without her efforts this book would
not be complete. I love you with all
my heart my angel Lia!

CONTENTS

DISCLAIMER 6

INTRODUCTION 7

WEAPON 1: Detect Signs, Symptoms and risk factors early 9

WEAPON 2: Don't procrastinate – Start fighting immediately! 12

WEAPON 3: Create inner "Mental Watcher" for early signs,
symptoms and risk factors of cold and flu 14

WEAPON 4: Activate all inner strength and willpower to
avoid sickness and recover quickly! 16

WEAPON 5: Drink hot tea or any other hot beverage
every two to three hours 18

WEAPON 6: Forgotten Grandma's way of fighting cold and flu 21

WEAPON 7: Sore throat gargle that really works! 23

WEAPON 8: Inhale steam from boiled hot water with oils 25

WEAPON 9: Source Naturals – Wellness Formula 27

WEAPON 10: Take vitamins and minerals supplements
to strengthen the immune system 29

WEAPON 11: Take B vitamins 40

WEAPON 12: Take raw ginger, turmeric and cayenne pepper 44

WEAPON 13: Take horseradish and garlic 47

WEAPON 14: Take rosehips, hibiscus, echinacea and elderberry 50

WEAPON 15: Drink apple cider vinegar with cayenne pepper,
cinnamon and lemon juice 53

WEAPON 16: Take medicinal mushrooms   56

WEAPON 17: Take vegan protein, glutamine and BCAA supplements   60

WEAPON 18: Take healthy fats — black seed, oregano, flaxseed and medium chain triglycerides (MCT) oils   63

WEAPON 19: Increase food intake   66

WEAPON 20: Take oranges, mandarins, tangerines and lemons with some peel   68

WEAPON 21: Eat a carrot and an apple every day   70

WEAPON 22: Berries   72

WEAPON 23: Eat more fruit   75

WEAPON 24: Vegetables and greens   79

WEAPON 25: Legumes, grains and seeds   83

WEAPON 26: Eat nuts   87

WEAPON 27: Avoid animal–based and highly processed foods high in sugar, bad fats and gluten   91

WEAPON 28: Rest as much as possible and get adequate sleep   95

WEAPON 29: Stay warm. Maintain good personal hygiene. Keep your body moving and exercise regularly. Avoid contact with people showing cold or flu symptoms.   98

FINAL THOUGHTS AND RECOMMENDATIONS   100

DISCLAIMER

This book is not professional medical advice and should not be used as such. Consult your doctor before following the advice in this book.

We are all different and while the remedies in this book are effective for most people, there is no guarantee that all methods below will work for everyone.

Some people may have allergies or have adverse reactions to some of the foods, vitamins and ingredients described.

Many of the methods described in this book are anecdotal in nature, and although they always work for me and many people I know, maybe they will not help you get better or recover from cold and flu.

Always seek additional professional medical help if your cold or flu symptoms do not improve after 3–5 days.

Consult a doctor if you decide to alter your diet and start new supplements and if you are unsure how your body will react to new foods and supplements. This is especially important if you are pregnant or breastfeeding.

Ask your doctor about safe dosages of new supplements and foods.
Never overdose on any vitamin, mineral or other supplement as this may be harmful to your health and even lead to potential organ failure or untimely passing.

Discuss your full medical history with your doctor before adding new vitamins, minerals or supplements to your diet. Ensure that you don't have pre–existing medical conditions as taking new vitamins, minerals or supplements can lead to worsening of health which can eventually cause irreversible harm.

Always read all instructions on labels of supplements.

This book is written as theoretical advice only. None of the statements in this book have been evaluated or endorsed by FDA (USA), TGA (Australia) or any similar governing body.

By using the advice in this book you thoroughly accept and agree that the author cannot be held liable and is not responsible for adverse effects, allergic reactions or other negative health issues that you may experience as a result of using advice offered in this book. By using the advice given in this book you accept and agree that the outcomes of using this book are your sole responsibility. Do not use the advice given in this book if you disagree with these disclaimers.

INTRODUCTION

First, I would like to thank you for purchasing this book. Your contribution will greatly help me to further research subjects on health and well–being.

I always believed that in some mysterious ways the books we are meant to read end up in our hands at the right time. And somehow you are reading these lines now, which may suggest that it is meant to be.

I am not a doctor by profession, but since a very early age I was interested, read and researched health and wellness topics as much as I could so I could make my life and the lives of people around me better in some ways.

It took more than ten years to discover, research, try and test the methods that actually prevent, relieve symptoms and help to shorten recovery times of cold and flu.

This book describes many methods that can prevent and decrease the duration of most cold and flu–related diseases.

It is in no way guaranteed that any of the methods described in this book will be effective against the novel COVID–19 coronavirus, which has turned our lives upside down in the recent months.

As of October 2020, there is no proven or guaranteed way to recover from this new virus. However, many methods in this book describe how to strengthen the immune system, which is our main hope and strongest available weapon to fight infections that take hold of our bodies.

So far it has been proven worldwide that patients with healthy immune systems and no underlying health conditions have a much better chance of recovery from COVID–19. So, taking great care and strengthening our body's natural immune system's defence mechanism is our only hope if we become infected with COVID–19.

The immune systems can fight disease quite effectively on their own if they have the necessary means.

In order to enable the immune system to perform at its peak, we need to create the necessary conditions. We need to be well rested and provide our bodies with the required vitamins, minerals, macro and micro nutrients for the immune system to fight any given disease.

Our bodies are finely balanced machines that must be in good shape to perform at their best and combat diseases naturally. Our role in this process is to provide the necessary resources so that our bodies can utilize their inner potential to combat illness.

I will start with my own story . . .

Around ten years ago I would get cold or flu–related diseases at least a few times a year. Each time my illness would last from one week to sometimes over 3 weeks, which made me unable to work as I felt very sick, weak and unmotivated to do anything other than stay home and "treat" myself. Almost every time when my cold or flu would last over one week I would go to a doctor and every time the solution would seem to be the same. I would be given paracetamol and antibiotics. The problem was that sometimes I did not feel better for another one or two weeks and I would feel down and lose weeks of productivity. After a while I could no longer accept that fact, and I started to look for solutions on how to fight and recover from cold and flu naturally. One by one, I read many books on this topic, researched and studied supplements, vitamins, herbs and natural remedies that people have used around the world for centuries, and as a result I gradually developed a cold– and flu–fighting system. For more than ten years it has helped me to prevent serious cold or flu sickness lasting more than three to five days, and I have very mild symptoms.

I'm not a doctor, nor am I a medical scientist. I simply constantly looked for, researched and tested one by one on myself methods and remedies related to curing diseases caused by cold and flu. Gradually, after trying many things, I selected only the ones that worked best for me and for most people around me.

I present my findings in the pages below. It took more than ten years to develop this step–by–step system to combat cold and flu, and I believe that anyone applying the strategies below can achieve similar results. Many of the methods and supplements described in this book are backed by years of collective scientific research with trials and tests performed by scientists worldwide to prove that certain supplement, vitamin, herb or other remedies are effective against cold and flu.

For best results the following methods and remedies must be used together. I highly recommend testing each one on yourself to see what works best for you, so you can always have disease fighting "weapons" in your arsenal should you detect the first signs of cold or flu.

I made this book as concise as possible so that the readers can start using the practical advice without poring through tiresome theoretical discussions.

Wish everyone the best of health. I hope these pages help you recover from cold or flu at a faster rate than before or prevent you from getting sick in the first place.

Presented below is the list of "Weapons" that can help you fight and kill cold– and flu–related illnesses in the shortest possible time.

DETECT SIGNS, SYMPTOMS AND RISK FACTORS EARLY

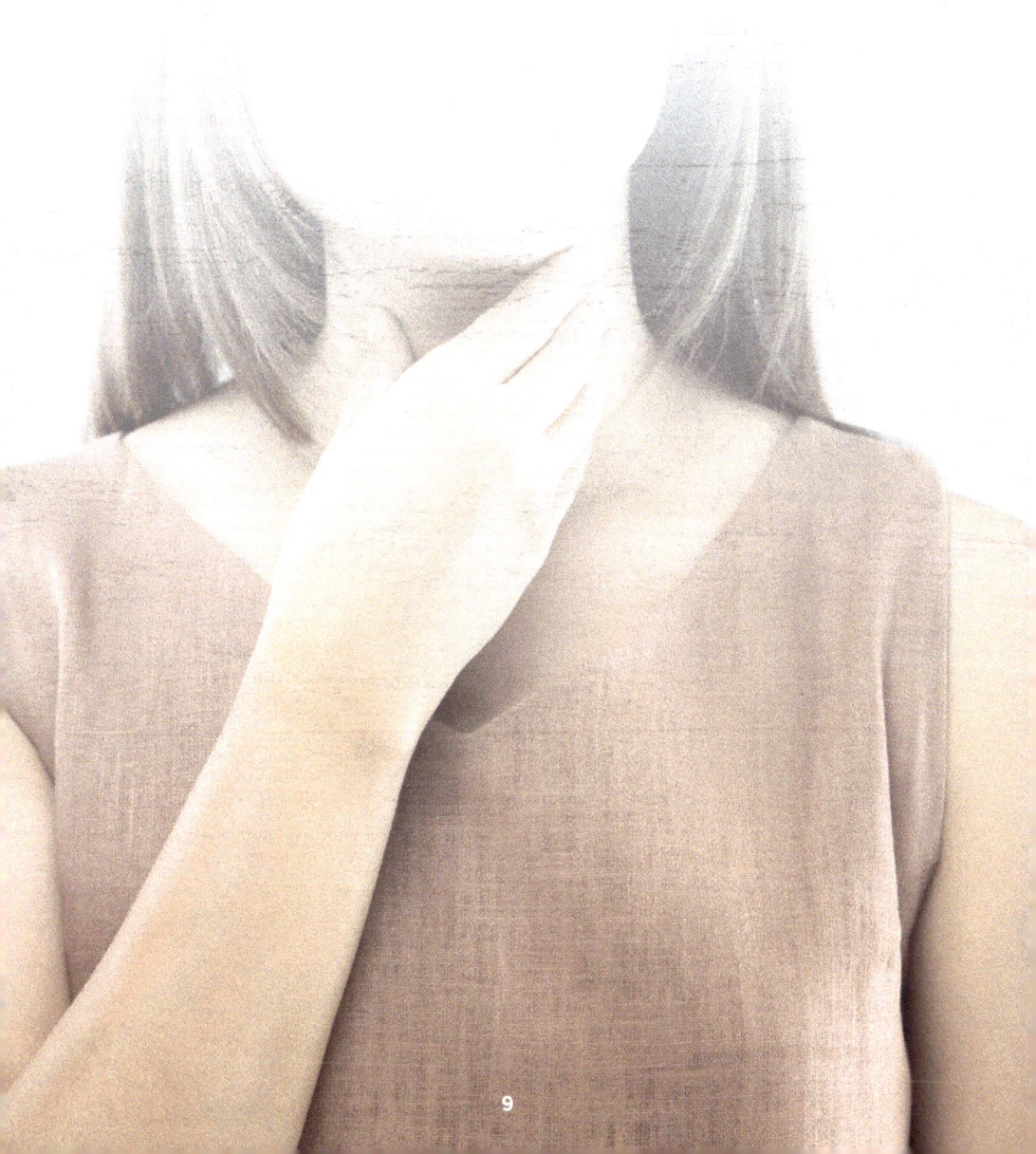

The most important step when preventing cold or flu is to detect the first signs, symptoms and risk factors of ill health early when you are not yet sick but may be at risk. It is important to act when you start feeling very mild symptoms.

The most common first signs and symptoms

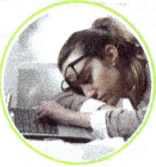

Feeling weak and tired
You may start feeling weak and tired for no apparent reason, even though you ate usual meals and slept well the night before.

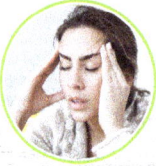

Unexplained headache
Feeling unexpected headache is often a sign that cold or flu is starting even though you don't yet have other more obvious symptoms.

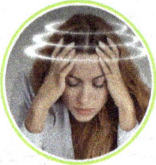

Dizziness
Feeling a bit dizzy is another sign of getting unwell that should sound an alarm.

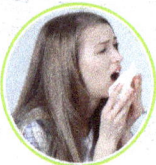

Sneezing
Sometimes you will randomly sneeze once or twice for no obvious reason. Maybe you accidentally inhaled dust or glanced at bright light, but it also may be that you are at the earliest stage of coming down with cold or flu.

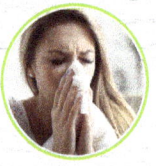

Runny nose
As with random sneezing, it may appear that your nose is slightly irritated and feels tickled inside as if you inhaled dust. Nonetheless, a runny nose is a definite sign that you may be getting cold or flu. Never let it pass unnoticed.

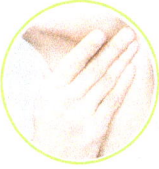

Itchy or slightly irritated throat
This is a common symptom if you are starting to get cold or flu. Your throat feels funny as if lightly tickled or itchy without being sore yet. You will feel as if something is in your throat without pain at this early stage.

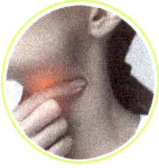

Sore throat
A sore throat that starts to feel more and more itchy is an obvious sign that you are coming down with cold or flu.

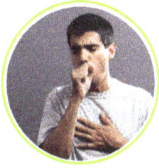

Coughing
Sometimes coughing randomly a couple of times may be a warning sign that soon you may get sick. This symptom should never be underestimated.

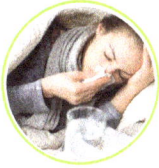

Suddenly feeling hot or cold in your body, head, hands or legs for no apparent reason
A possible sign that you are getting invaded by cold or flu.

Some signs that you may have a higher risk of getting cold or flu and need to start fighting and take immediate action include

1. Your body gets really cold when you are out. Especially if your feet, neck and throat get very cold for a prolonged period of time.

2. You eat a lot of ice–cream, cold or frozen foods or drink one or more large cold beverages.

3. You are exposed to a cold wind or breeze for prolonged period of time;

4. You are in contact with one or more people who look like they might suffer from cold or flu.

5. You don't eat or sleep well for one or more days.

6. You do too much physical exercise and feel tired or lethargic for a long time after exercising – strenuous exercise programs deplete the body of many important macro and micro nutrients and weaken the immune systems for a while, which can make it much easier to get sick with cold or flu.

DON'T PROCRASTINATE – START FIGHTING IMMEDIATELY!

Don't be lazy and procrastinate even for thirty minutes if you have detected a sign, symptom or risk factor from chapter one. Delay may cost an extra few days of tiresome recovery efforts to get well again!

You should make sure to always start fighting the cold or flu immediately if you detect a sign, symptom or risk factor. Even if you are not actually getting cold and flu but feel you are at risk, you can still apply the methods below as a precaution with no negative effects.

I will repeat – it is extremely important to "catch" the first signs or symptoms and act immediately. Sometimes even a short delay of one or two hours will let the cold– or flu–related infection get a good hold of our bodies making it much harder to fight off and achieve full recovery.

I highly recommend memorizing the signs, symptoms and risk factors from chapter one. If you find it hard to remember, write them on a piece of paper that you can keep nearby and read them once a day so you are always ready to take immediate action.

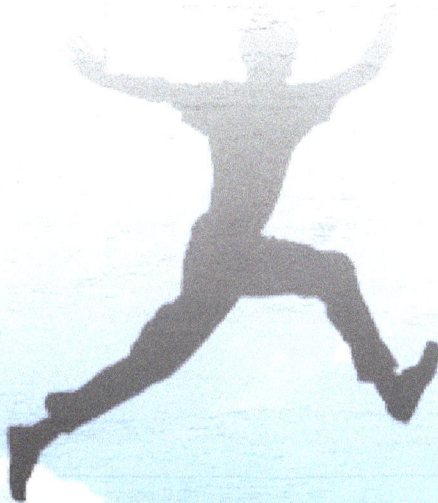

WEAPON 3

CREATE INNER "MENTAL WATCHER" FOR EARLY SIGNS, SYMPTOMS AND RISK FACTORS OF COLD AND FLU

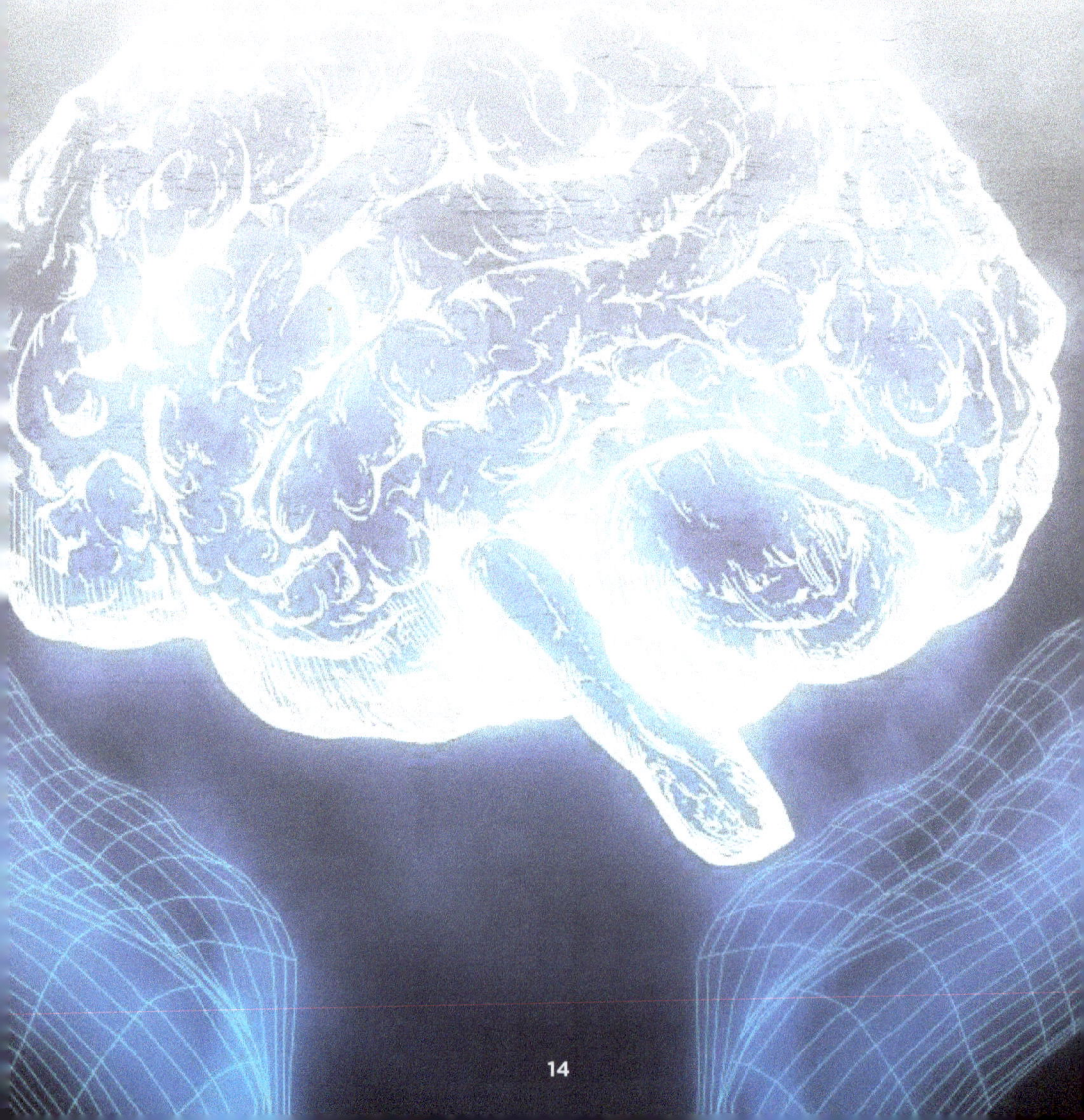

This technique requires a good deal of mental effort and some perseverance on our part. We can actually install an imaginary mental watcher in our mind if we practice this technique on a daily basis for at least sixty to ninety days.

Everyone can do it as it takes only a couple of minutes about three times a day. For best results it should be done at least once in the morning, once around midday and once before you go to sleep.

Here is the method

Imagine that somewhere above your head there is an invisible conscious being that is constantly alert and on a lookout for the early symptoms and risk factors of getting sick with cold or flu as described in chapter one. You can make this entity anything you like – a cat, a dog, a bird or any favourite character from movies – just make sure that the image of this watcher is memorable and vivid and you can imagine it at any time. Keep imagining your chosen character floating somewhere above your head for a couple of minutes. Try to visualize it as if you can even touch it. Make it as real and as vivid as possible.

Next – armour your watcher with the symptoms and risk factors – for another few minutes keep repeating the early signs, symptoms and risk factors of getting sick described in chapter one and keep asking your watcher to always sound a loud alarm of your choice if it detects a dangerous sign. The alarm may be a voice, a ringing bell or anything you prefer, but make sure that it will get your attention and push you to take immediate action.

The purpose of this technique is to make sure that you always remember the early signs and symptoms and are always ready to take action without delay.

I prefer to do this technique with closed eyes in a calm, quiet place. But with practice it can be done anywhere, even in noisy surroundings and in bright daylight.

WEAPON 4

ACTIVATE ALL INNER STRENGTH AND WILLPOWER TO AVOID SICKNESS AND RECOVER QUICKLY!

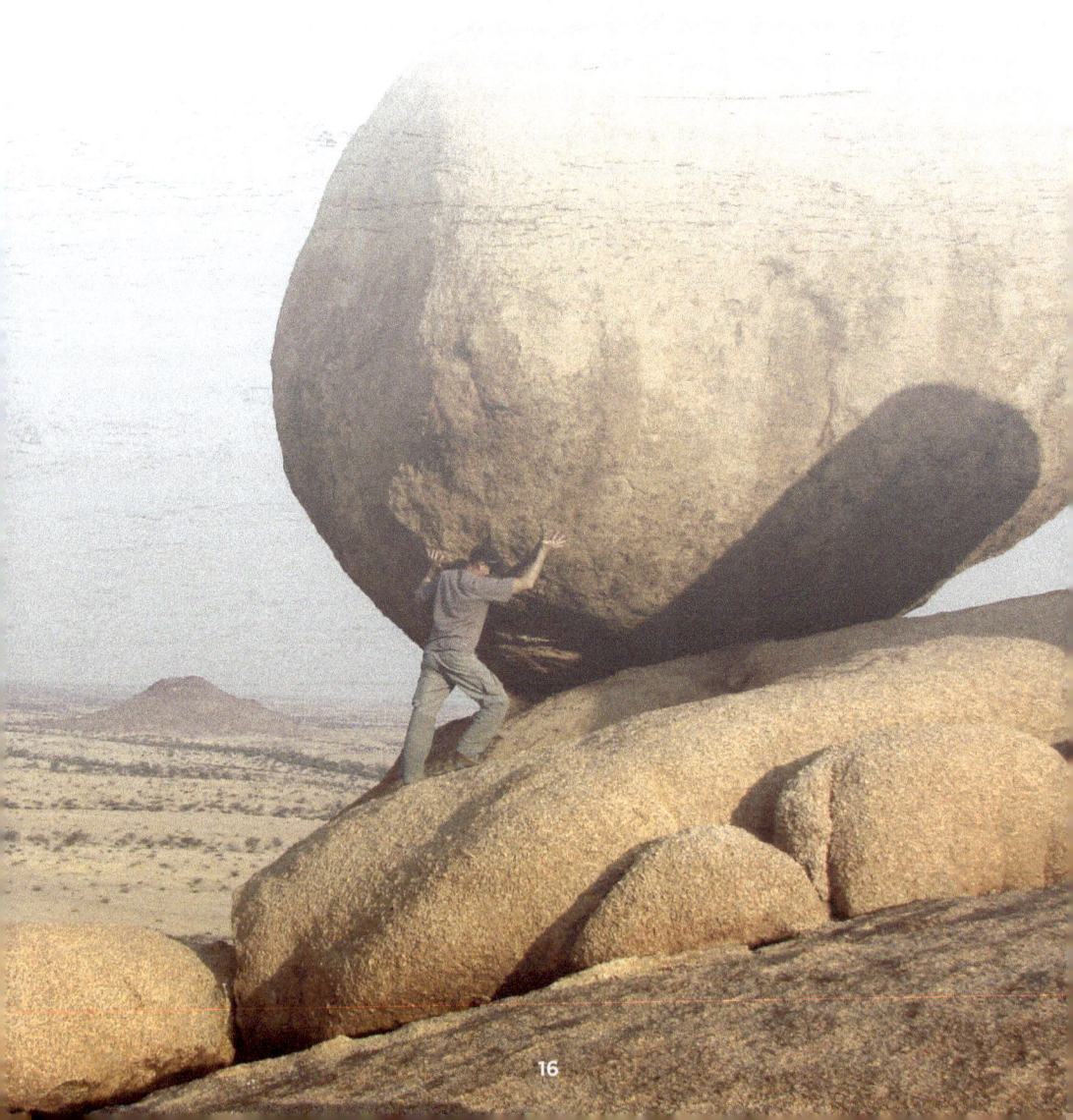

Inner determination and willpower play a huge part in the recovery process.

Always stay positive and never give up fighting however bad you may feel and believe with absolute conviction that you will recover as soon as possible.

Apart from meeting all purely physical demands of our bodies, we must also ensure that our mental attitude is "tuned" correctly to fight disease. This can be achieved via cultivating strong inner conviction and belief that you will recover from the disease in the shortest time possible. This belief must be consistent and without any hesitation or doubts. All willpower must be summoned to support the belief that this is a short–time flu or cold and that you will recover in a matter of one or two days at most. You should always be in active "fight" mode mentally with the strength of your inner will urging your body and immune system to constantly kill the disease minute by minute. You must imagine and feel as if you have already recovered and that your body is healthy, strong and full of the necessary resources to quickly fight off any disease.

You have to sincerely want to get better. Focus all the strength of your inner drive and your willpower. This will enable your body to switch into the best possible mode for fighting the illness.

Numerous successful scientific studies prove that even placebo and water work much better with a positive mindset and a belief in quick recovery when compared to people who are hesitant, scared and do not want to recover or do not believe that they will get better.

Our minds and the strength of our willpower can almost create miracles if only we could learn to tune them to perform at their best.

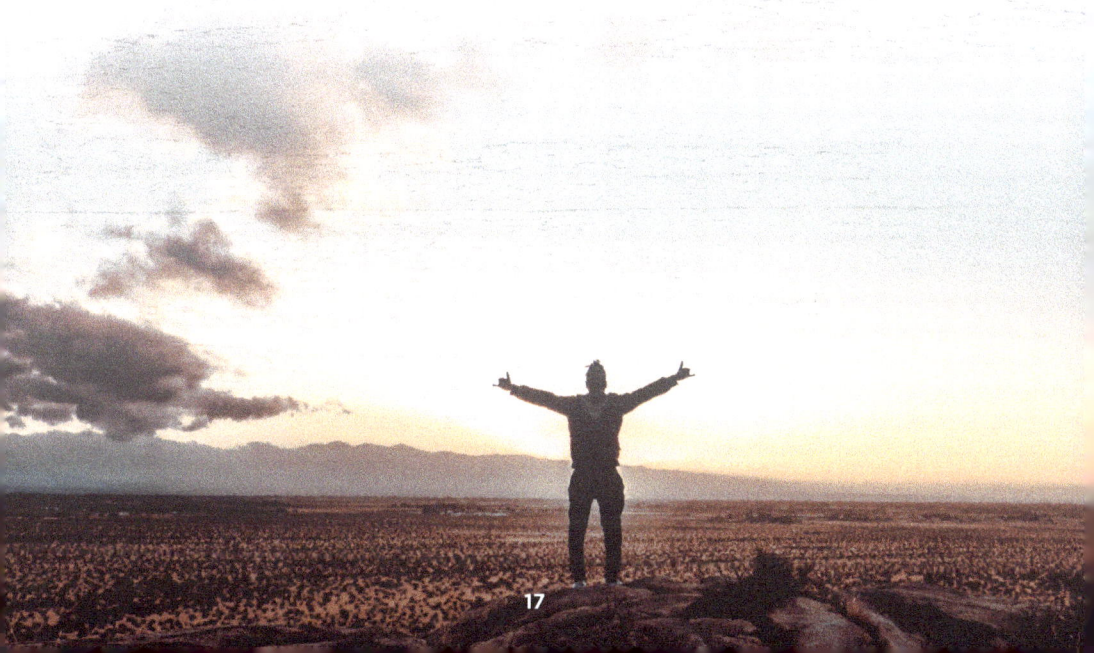

WEAPON 5

DRINK HOT TEA OR ANY OTHER HOT BEVERAGE EVERY TWO TO THREE HOURS

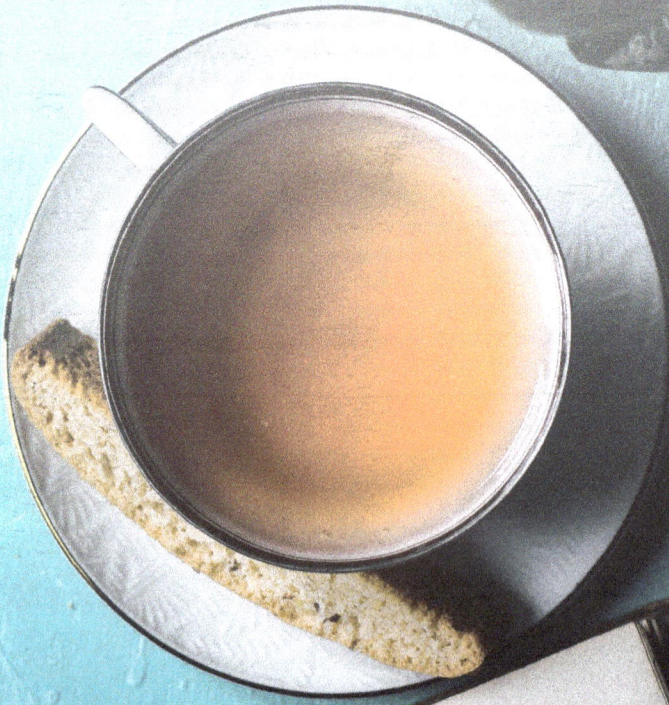

Keeping your body warm from inside by drinking hot teas and hot beverages every two to three hours is one of the most effective ways to fight cold and flu. Most cold and flu infections cannot survive high temperatures and hot environments so you should ensure that your body is always "hotter" than it usually is by drinking hot drinks at least once every two to three hours while you are experiencing symptoms or trying to prevent getting sick.

Some of my favorite recipes for hot drinks

Echinacea, rosehip, hibiscus, ginger, turmeric, raspberry jam and lemon cold– and flu–fighting tea:
Into one cup of boiling hot water add about one half teaspoon or more of grated raw ginger root, a half teaspoon or more of grated raw turmeric, 1 teaspoon of dried echinacea herb, half to one teaspoon of cut and sifted hibiscus, half to one teaspoon of cut and sifted rosehips, 1 teaspoon or more of raspberry jam, squeeze the juice from a slice of lemon and place the squeezed slice into the cup as well. Cover the cup with a small plate and let it steep for about three to five minutes. Drink a cup of this tea gradually while it's still hot every two to three hours throughout the day while you are having cold– or flu–related symptoms or use as a preventative measure.

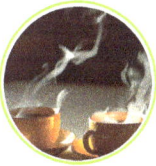

Gunpowder version of cold and flu fighting tea:
My favorite morning hot drink includes a mix of a half level teaspoon of dried gunpowder green tea, half teaspoon of dried hibiscus flowers, half teaspoon of dried rosehips and almost a full teaspoon of echinacea. Add ingredients to a large mug of boiling water and wait for at least five minutes before drinking. Apart from helping fight off cold or flu, this drink can also make you feel alert and adds a general sense of clarity and well–being.

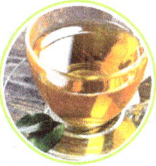

Coffee that makes you feel great and fights cold and flu:
Add a half teaspoon of quality ground coffee and half to one tablespoon of C8 MCT oil (caprylic acid) to the mug of hot water. Cover and let it steep for a few minutes. Drink while it's still hot. This coffee drink will make you feel great, alert and energized for at least a couple of hours.

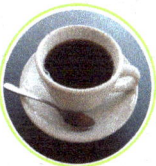

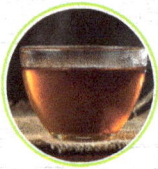

"Before bed" version of cold– and flu–fighting tea

For a better night's sleep while still fighting cold or flu, add a teaspoon of raspberry jam, a small pinch of ashwagandha herb powder, a teaspoon of dried chamomile flowers and half teaspoon of valerian roots to a medium–sized mug half–filled with hot water. Cover the mug for a few minutes and drink slowly while the tea is still hot. Don't fill the mug more than half full as drinking too much liquid before bed may cause a wakeful night.

You can make hot drinks with pretty much anything you like. You can brew a teabag of any herbal or non–herbal tea of your choice; add a teaspoon or less of jam or any herb to a large mug of boiling water. Or you can mix teas, herbs and fruits or fruit jams to create something unique and enjoyable.

For maximum cold– and flu–fighting benefits, drink at least one large mug of your favorite hot brew every two to three hours, and you will be well rewarded by recovering from your cold or flu much faster than usual.

Always make sure that your drinks are still hot while you are drinking them and always drink them slowly so you don't burn yourself.

Caffeine warning

Don't overuse caffeine and avoid caffeine after 2 pm as it may keep you awake, interfere with the quality of your sleep and have a negative effect on the immune system which in turn makes it hard to fight off the cold or flu.

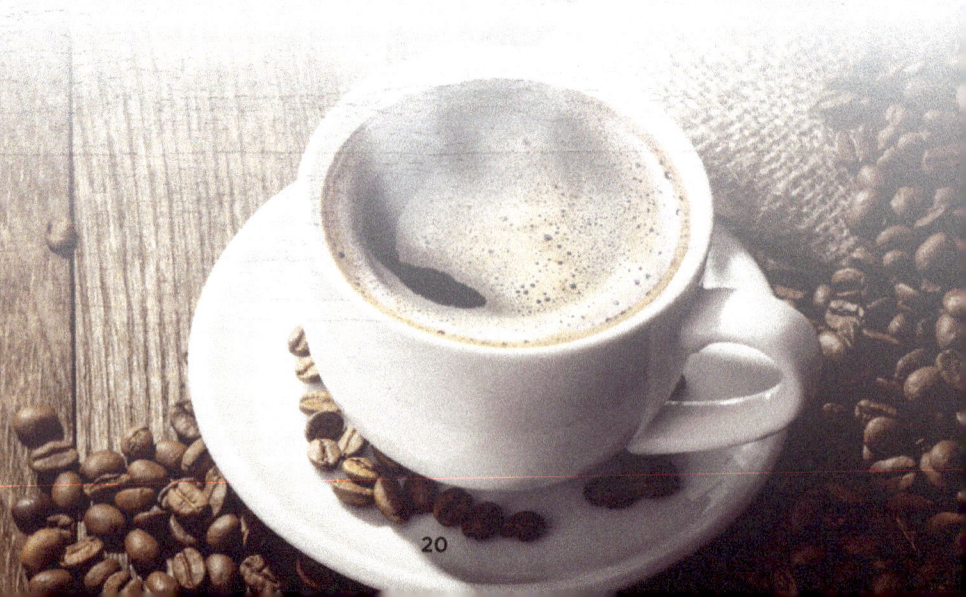

WEAPON 6

FORGOTTEN GRANDMA'S WAY OF FIGHTING COLD AND FLU

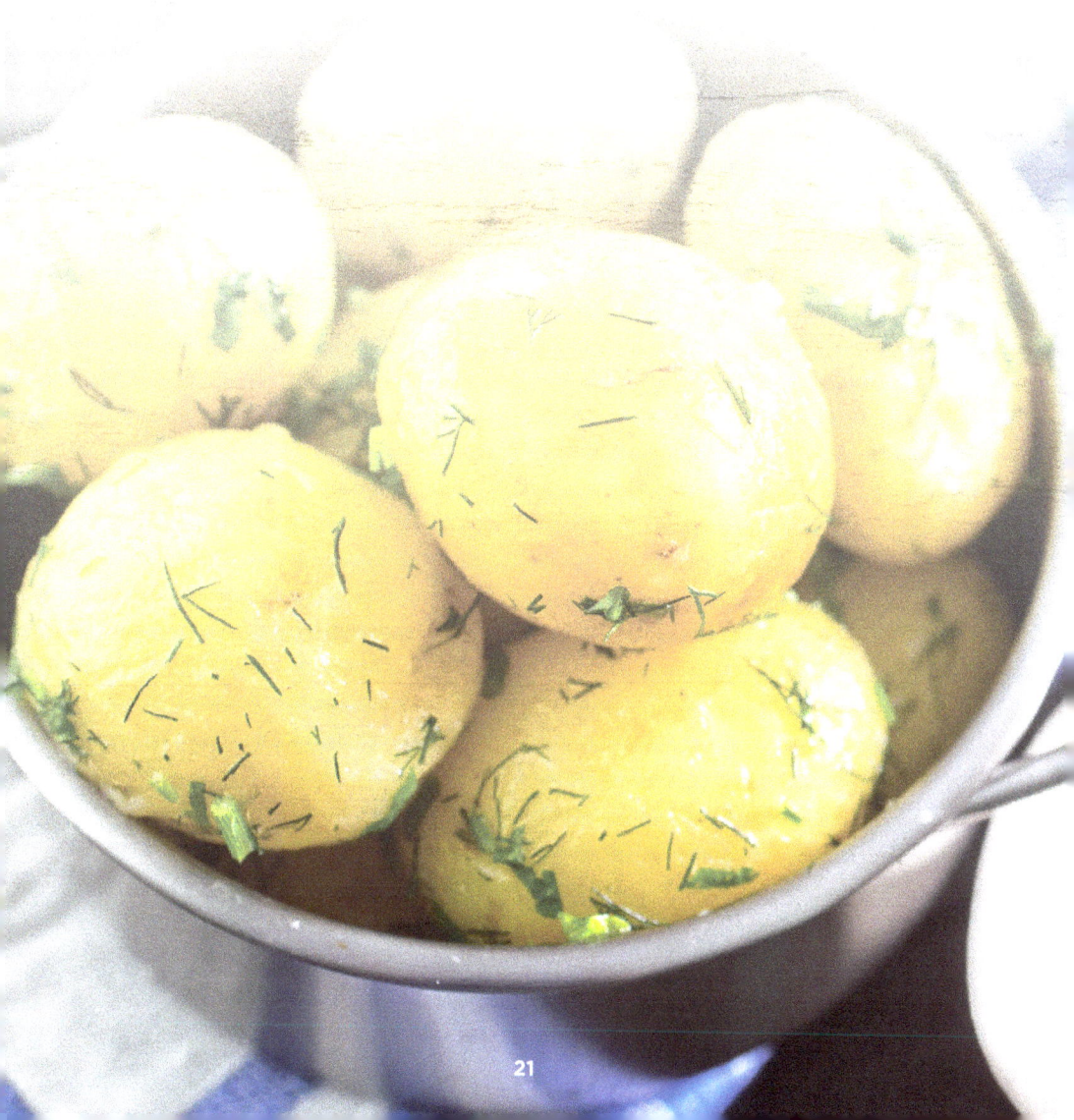

About eleven years ago I had a cold that lasted over two months and constantly made me feel down and sick with sore throat, runny nose, cough and high temperature. I have tried many cold and flu medicines available at the pharmacies, have gone to three doctors who prescribed lots of Panadol and three lengthy courses of antibiotics with no result. I could not recover no matter what and was eventually unable to work. At the end of the second month of being sick with that–most likely–a virus–related infection, I started to lose all hope of recovery. I told one of my friends about my situation and she suggested that I try this old "Boiled Potatoes" Ukrainian method from her grandma. I started applying it that night and after a few days, I started to experience noticeable progress and I recovered almost completely within about a week. At that time, I did not know about Source Naturals Wellness Formula, so maybe I would have recovered much quicker if I also took that formula. But none–the–less this method saved me that year.

Using this method

Boil two to three large potatoes in water until they become soft and mushy. Remove them from the water, mash them while they are hot and place the mashed paste in two to three plastic bags and make sure there are no leaks. Wrap the three plastic bags with at least two to three or more layers of a soft fabric or towels. Make sure that the fabric or towels are very warm but not too hot so you don't burn yourself. Lie down and place the wrapped potato paste around the chest, throat and neck areas. Cover yourself with a warm blanket and hold the hot potato paste on your body for at least thirty to forty–five minutes until the potatoes become colder than body temperature. Do this at least once a day before going to sleep at night. For better and more effective results, you can repeat this process three times a day—first thing in the morning, around midday and at night.

Warning

Don't burn yourself!

Be careful when handling hot potatoes. Never touch them with your hands. Use a large spoon and a potato masher to mash them and to move the hot potato paste into plastic bags. Take extra care also when wrapping these plastic bags with hot potatoes in fabric. You can use an extra towel or gloves to avoid burns. Make sure that the wrapped hot potato paste does not feel too hot when you place it on your chest, neck and throat. It should be very warm but not burning hot. Remove hot potatoes from your body immediately if you experience any discomfort.

WEAPON 7

SORE THROAT GARGLE THAT REALLY WORKS!

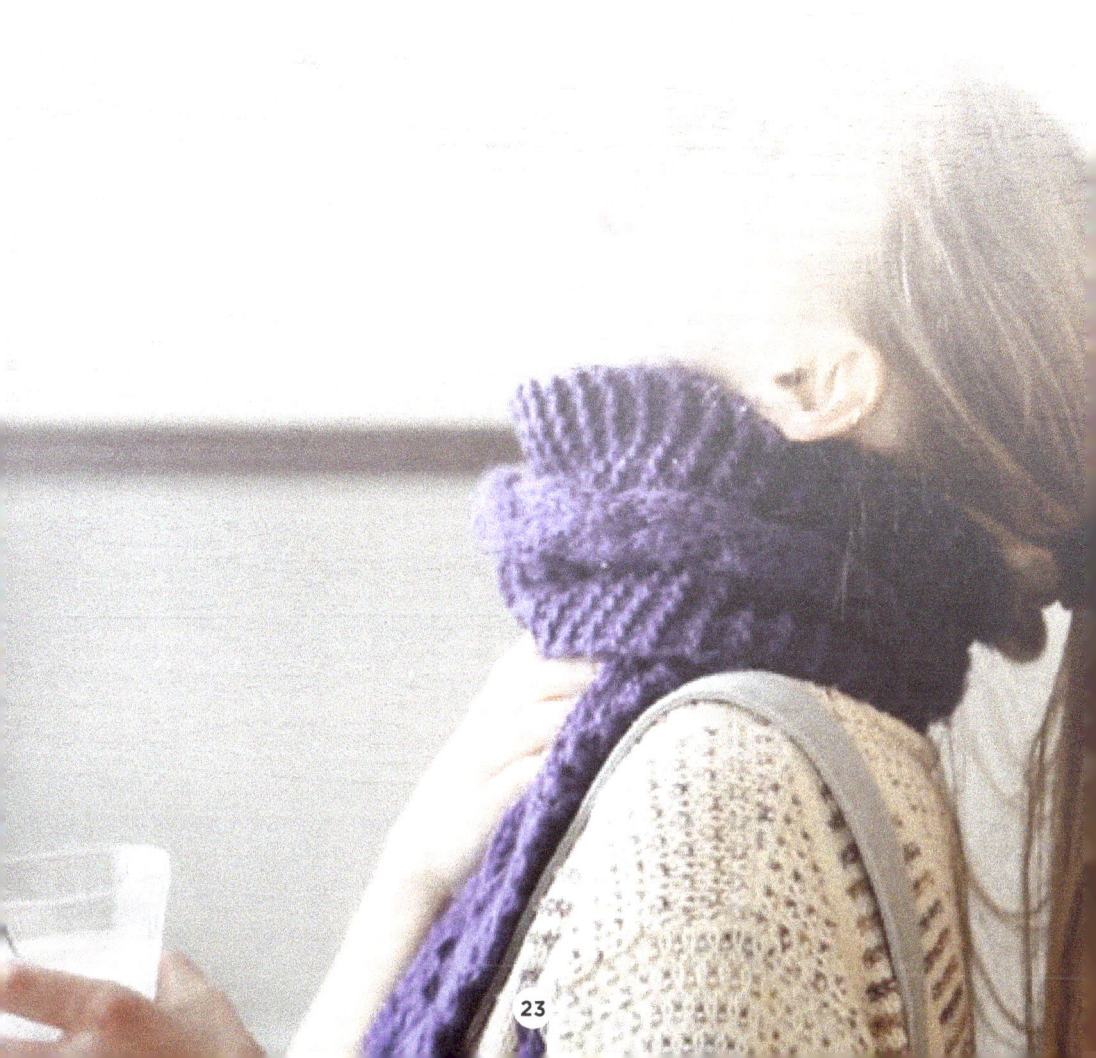

When I was recovering from a lengthy cold, which I described in the previous chapter, I also regularly gargled with salt, soda and eucalyptus oil.

Using the gargle solution described below is very effective and can help you get rid of sore throat and quickly recover from cold and flu. This method involves applying anti–viral and anti–bacterial agents directly to affected areas in your mouth.

Using this method

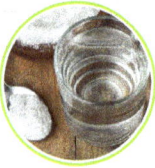

Add one teaspoon of salt, one teaspoon of soda bicarbonate and one to three small drops of eucalyptus oil to a large mug of warm water. Mix it well until salt and soda are dissolved.

Gargle with the solution at least once every couple of hours for thirty seconds or a bit longer every day until three days after all symptoms of sore throat disappear.

Yes, it sounds like a lot of gargling, but it is a very effective method to quickly get rid of cold and flu symptoms like sore throat or runny nose.

You can also try Betadine sore throat gargle – it is a 10 mg/ml solution of povidone–iodine (equivalent to 1 mg/ml of available iodine). It also works well for sore throat symptoms but is not recommended for frequent use as iodine can be harmful to the body. It should especially be avoided by people who are sensitive or allergic to iodine.

Warning

Before starting this method, consult your doctor to ensure you are not sensitive or allergic to the ingredients of the sore throat gargles described above.

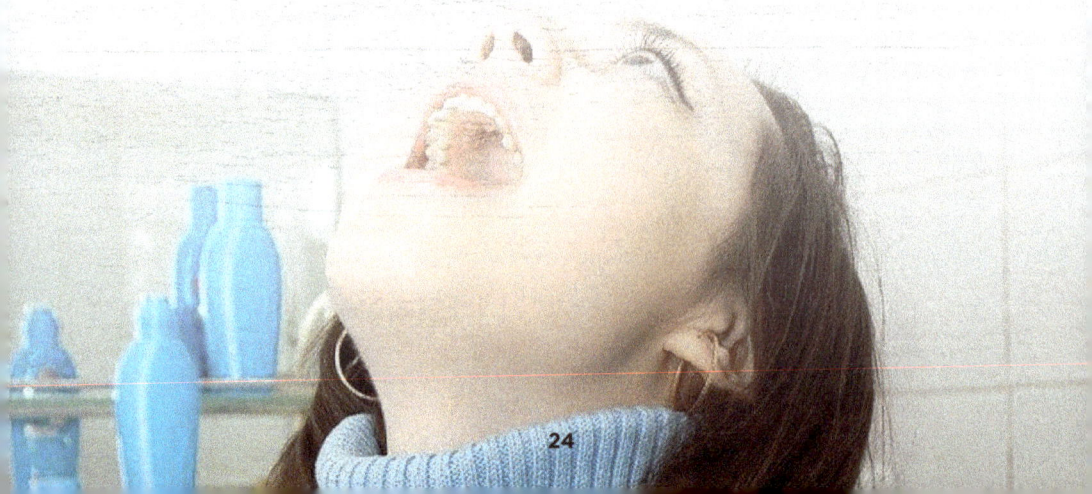

WEAPON 8

INHALE STEAM FROM BOILED HOT WATER WITH OILS

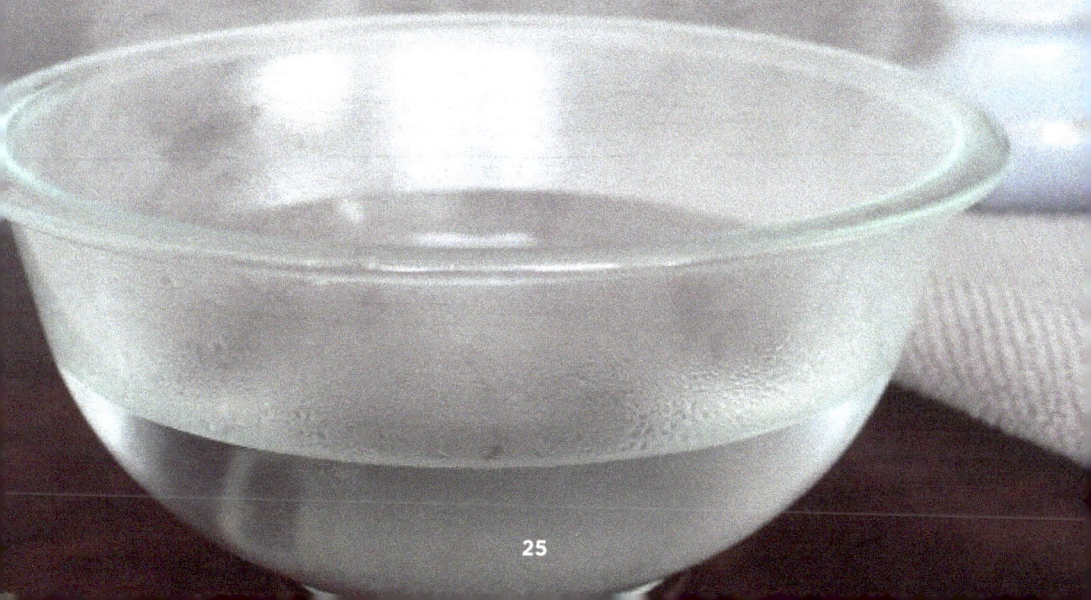

Using a steam inhaler regularly is another great weapon to implement when fighting cold or flu.

Some benefits of using a steam inhaler: helps you breathe easier and feel better by clearing nasal, trachea and bronchial passages; can kill cold– or flu–related infections by raising temperature levels in the respiratory tract. Inhalant oils have anti–viral and anti–bacterial properties which may further assist with killing cold– and flu–related infections in the respiratory tract.

Warning

Do not burn yourself when using a steam inhaler!

Be careful when using a steam inhaler to avoid burning the skin and respiratory tract. Always read the manual and follow the instructions. Do not overfill your inhaler with hot water, keep a safe distance when inhaling and avoid spilling hot water on your body.

Using this method

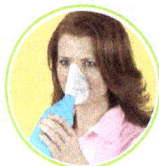

Add hot water to your inhaler according to the manufacturer's recommended level – *do not overfill your inhaler as it may cause you to burn yourself by spilling excess water on your body. Too much hot water can also make inhaling steam too hot which can lead to respiratory system burns.*

Add a few drops of mixed inhalant oils to the hot water inside the inhaler, stir it well to let the oils dissolve, and breathe the warm steam coming out of the inhaler for at least 6 to 10 minutes or longer at least 3 to 5 times a day. Make sure that you inhale through both the nose and the mouth. For the first 3 to 5 minutes, inhale through the nose only and then through the mouth only until you are done.

You can use a steam inhaler filled only with hot water, but for maximum effectiveness I highly recommend adding a few drops of mixed inhalant oils or at least a couple of drops of eucalyptus oil. Those oils have many cold– and flu–fighting and immune–system–boosting benefits which will help relieve symptoms and speed the recovery process.

Where to purchase a steam inhaler and inhalant oils

You can purchase a good steam inhaler at your local pharmacy, retail store, or online.

WEAPON 9

SOURCE NATURALS –
WELLNESS FORMULA

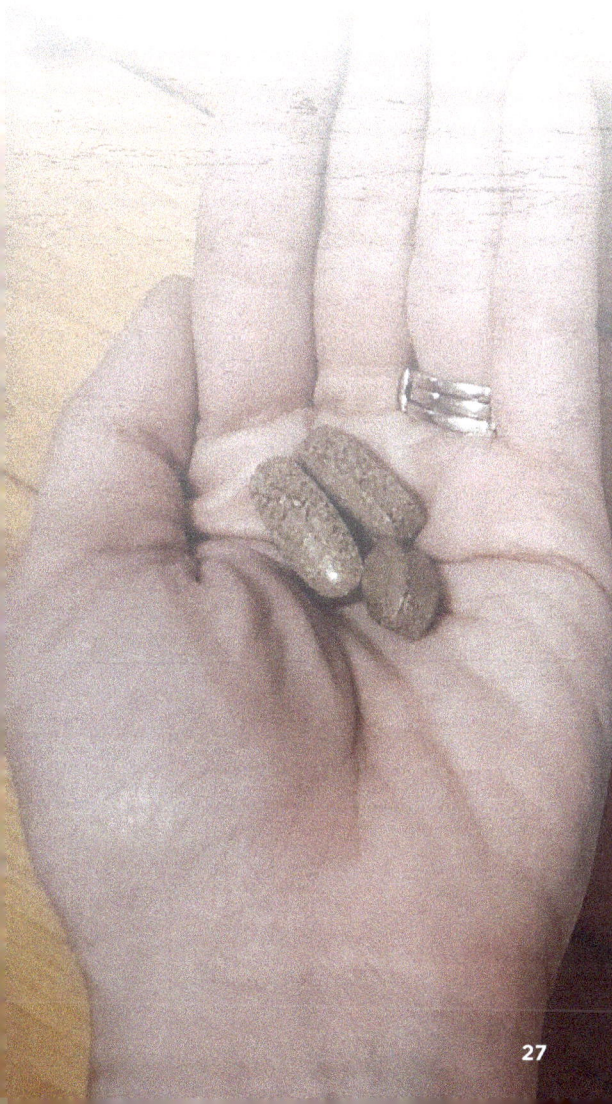

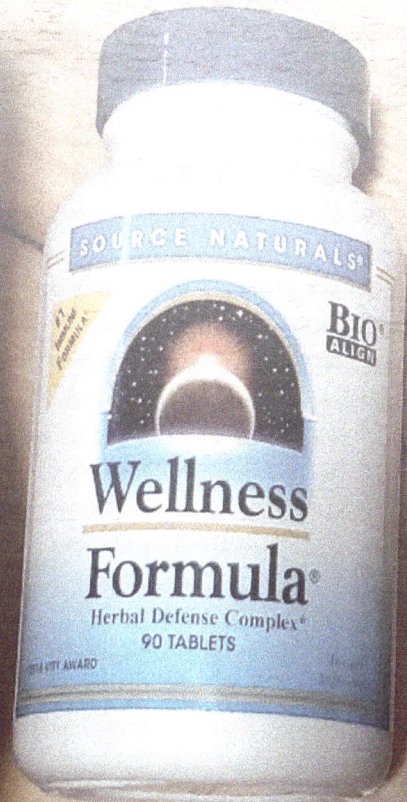

Wellness Formula by Source Naturals is a very effective supplement for strengthening the immune system.

It has great proportions of vitamins A, C, D–3, zinc, selenium and copper. This supplement also has a host of other immune supporting natural ingredients that work in synergy so that your body can fight off cold or flu as quickly as possible.

It is by far the best supplement I have taken for cold and flu. It has always helped me recover in a couple of days instead of weeks. Thousands of people have confirmed its high potency and effectiveness over the years. Many people say that by taking Wellness Formula alone they were able to fight off cold or flu–related illnesses much faster than by using other methods.

It can be bought online and in local health stores.

Best way to take Wellness Formula

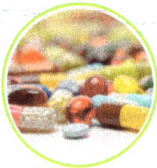

For the very first mild symptoms, or as a preventive measure when you think you may be at risk of getting cold or flu, take 2 tablets in the morning and then 1 tablet every 2–3 hours until all symptoms completely disappear.

For moderate symptoms, when you are developing a sore throat and runny nose or high fever, take 3 tablets in the morning and then 2 tablets every 3 hours until all symptoms are gone. For more aggressive cold and flu infections that quickly develop a bad sore throat, high fever, runny nose, coughs and general fatigue, take 3 tablets in the morning and then 2–3 tablets every 3 hours as recommended on the manufacturer's label.

In the past five plus years, Wellness Formula always worked like "magic" for me and helped me recover in a matter of 1 to a few days at most from cold or flu symptoms. I cannot recommend this supplement highly enough.

As with any supplement, please consult your doctor before taking it. Make sure that you are not allergic to any ingredients, especially if you have pre–existing medical conditions or if you are pregnant or breastfeeding.

WEAPON 10

TAKE VITAMINS AND MINERALS SUPPLEMENTS TO STRENGTHEN THE IMMUNE SYSTEM

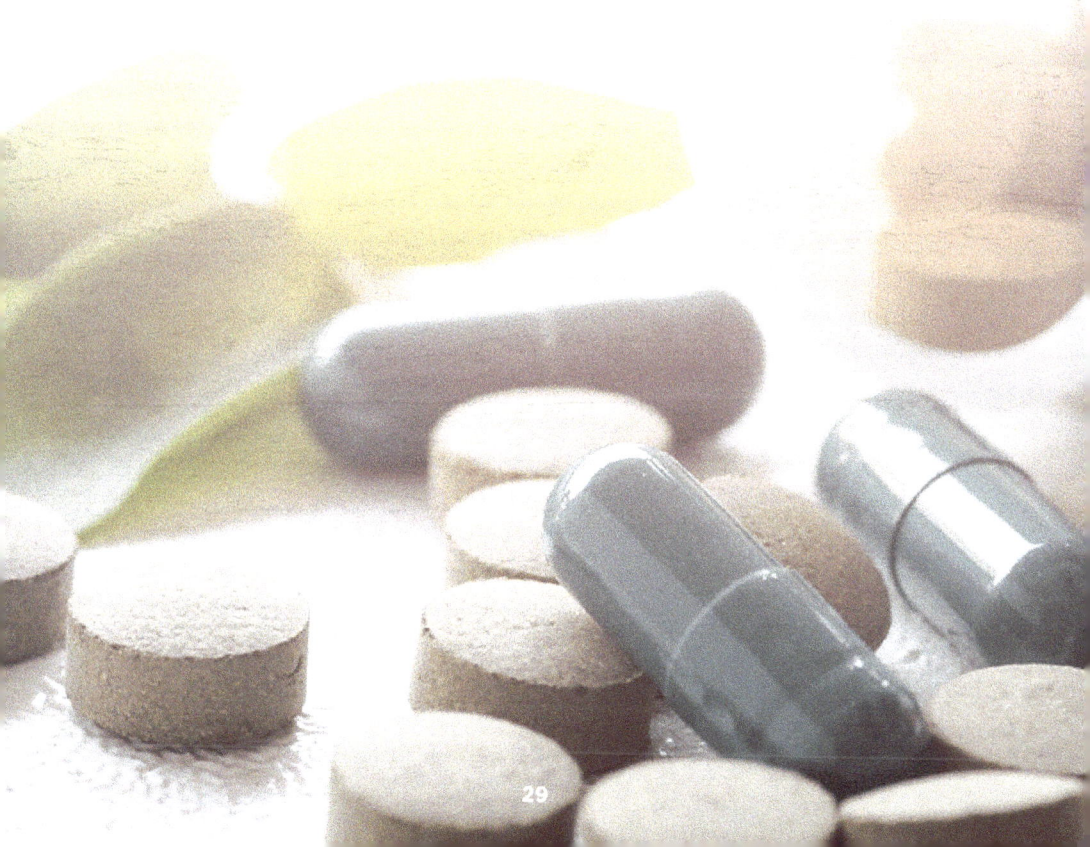

If you can't acquire the Wellness Formula described in the previous chapter, you can take vitamins A, C, D3, zinc, selenium and copper separately instead.

Warning

Don't take the vitamins and minerals listed in this chapter if you are taking Wellness Formula as it contains all these vitamins in good proportions and dosages. Stop taking Wellness Formula if you prefer to take vitamins and minerals separately. This is very important as overdosing with vitamins and minerals can be very harmful for your overall health and can lead to eventual organ failure.

It is highly recommended to test both methods. First take Wellness Formula for a while and see how it works; then stop taking it and take all the vitamins and minerals described below instead of taking Wellness Formula and see how they work for you. Eventually, choose what worked better, what made you feel better and helped you recover from cold or flu faster.

How to take vitamins and minerals

For best results split the tablets into 4 or 6 parts and take a small piece of each tablet every 3–4 hours so you maintain consistent levels of the vitamins and minerals in your bloodstream to enable the immune system to fight the disease without interruption.

Vitamin A

Vitamin A is a potent antioxidant that our bodies need for eye and vision health, for the reproductive system, fetal development, and most importantly for proper functioning of the immune system. Vitamin A is best taken in combination of beta–carotene and palmitate forms.

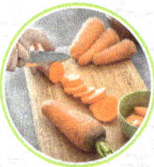

Directions

Take at least 3000 IU or beta–carotene and 2000 IU of palmitate form of vitamin A throughout the day. When you have more severe symptoms of cold or flu up to 15000 IU of beta–carotene and 10000 IU of palmitate can be taken in separate smaller doses during the day.

Natural sources of vitamin A

If you can't get a good source or vitamin A as a supplement in tablet form, you can always enrich your diet with the natural foods listed below. They are rich in vitamin A:

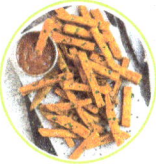

Sweet Potato (cooked)
1 cup: 1,836 mcg (204% DV)
1,043 mcg per 100 grams (116% DV)

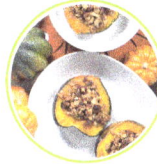

Winter Squash (cooked)
1 cup: 1,144 mcg (127% DV)
558 mcg per 100 grams (62% DV)

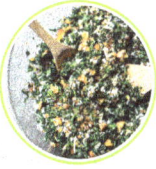

Kale (cooked)
1 cup: 885 mcg (98% DV)
681 mcg per 100 grams (76% DV)

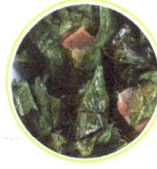

Collards (cooked)
1 cup: 722 mcg (80% DV)
380 mcg per 100 grams (42% DV)

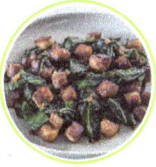

Turnip Greens (cooked)
1 cup: 549 mcg (61% DV)
381 mcg per 100 grams (42% DV)

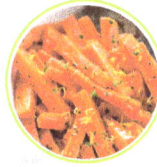

Carrot (cooked)
1 medium carrot: 392 mcg (44% DV)
381 mcg per 100 grams (42% DV)

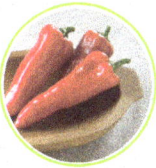

Sweet Red Pepper (raw)
1 large pepper: 257 mcg (29% DV)
157 mcg per 100 grams (17% DV)

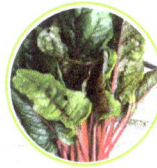

Swiss Chard (raw)
1 leaf: 147 mcg (16% DV)
306 mcg per 100 grams (34% DV)

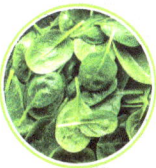

Spinach (raw)
1 cup: 141 mcg (16% DV)
469 mcg per 100 grams (52% DV)

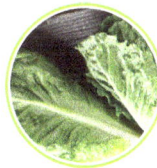

Romaine Lettuce (raw)
1 large leaf: 122 mcg (14% DV)
436 mcg per 100 grams (48% DV).

Vitamin C

Vitamin C is a very powerful antioxidant that strengthens the immune system. It is involved in production of lymphocytes and phagocytes (white blood cells) that help our bodies fight infection. Vitamin C also enhances the effectiveness of these white blood cells and protects them from damage by free radicals. Vitamin C accumulates in the skin to strengthen the protective barrier. Pneumonia patients who take higher doses of vitamin C usually have much shorter recovery times. It is one of the best vitamins to take if you need to make the immune system more efficient at fighting cold– or flu–related disease.

Vitamin C is best taken in the form of ascorbic acid crystals.

Dosage

Vitamin C is generally safe to take in high doses. For best results take 800 mg to 1500 mg every 2–3 hours while you have cold and flu symptoms or as a preventive measure when you are at risk of getting sick. Take 300 mg to 500 mg every 3 hours for up to 3 to 5 days after full recovery.

Natural sources of vitamin C

If you can't get vitamin C in tablet or powder form, you can always consume foods listed below that naturally contain high amounts:

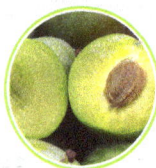

Kakadu plums
One plum: 481 mg
of vitamin C
5,300 mg per 100 grams (530% DV)

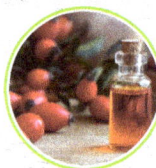

Rose hips
Approximately six pieces of this fruit deliver 132% of the DV
426 mg per 100 grams

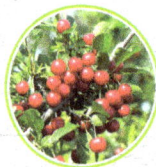

Red acerola cherries (Malpighia emarginata)
One–half cup (49 grams) delivers 822 mg of vitamin C, 913% of the DV

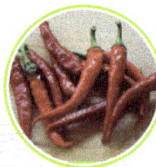

Chili peppers
one green chili pepper 109 mg – 121% DV
One red chili pepper – 65 mg – 72% DV
242 mg per 100 grams

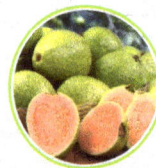

Guava – One guava 126 mg of vitamin C – 140% of the DV
228 mg per 100 grams

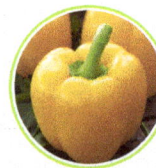

Sweet yellow peppers
one–half cup (75 grams) – 137 mg – 152% of the DV
181 mg per 100 grams

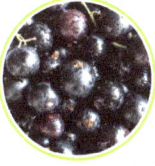

Blackcurrants – One–half cup (56 grams) – 101 mg – 112% DV 183 mg per 100 grams

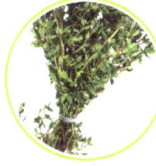

Thyme (fresh) – One ounce (28 grams) – 45 mg – 50% DV 160 mg per 100 grams

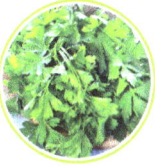

Parsley (fresh) – Two tablespoons (8 grams) – 10 mg – 11% DV 133 mg per 100 grams

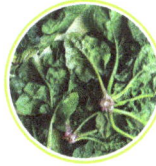

Mustard Spinach (raw) – one cup – 195 mg – 217% of the DV

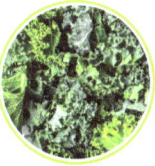

Kale 80 – One cup (raw) – 80 mg – 89% DV One cup (cooked) – 53 mg – 59% DV 120 mg per 100 grams

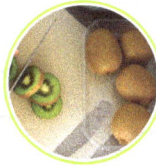

Kiwi – One medium kiwi – 71 mg – 79% DV 93 mg per 100 grams

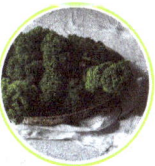

Broccoli – One–half cup (cooked) – 51 mg – 57% DV 89 mg per 100 grams

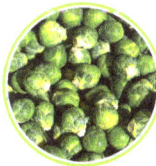

Brussels Sprouts – One–half cup (cooked) – 49 mg – 54% DV 85 mg per 100 grams

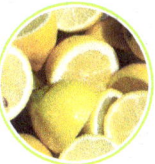

Lemons – One medium size lemon (Raw with peel) – 83 mg – 92% DV 77 mg per 100 grams

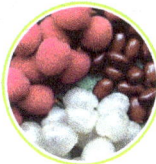

Lychees – one–cup – 151% DV 72 mg per 100 grams

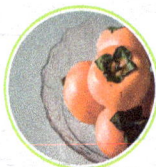

American persimmon (whole) – 16.5 mg – 18% DV
66 mg per 100 grams

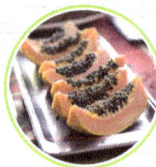

Papayas – One cup (145 grams) – 87 mg – 97% DV
62 mg per 100 grams

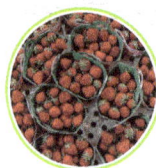

Strawberries one cup (152 grams) – 89 mg – 99% DV
59 mg per 100 grams

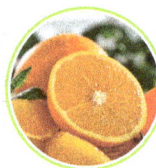

Oranges – One medium orange – 70 mg – 78% DV
53 mg per 100 grams

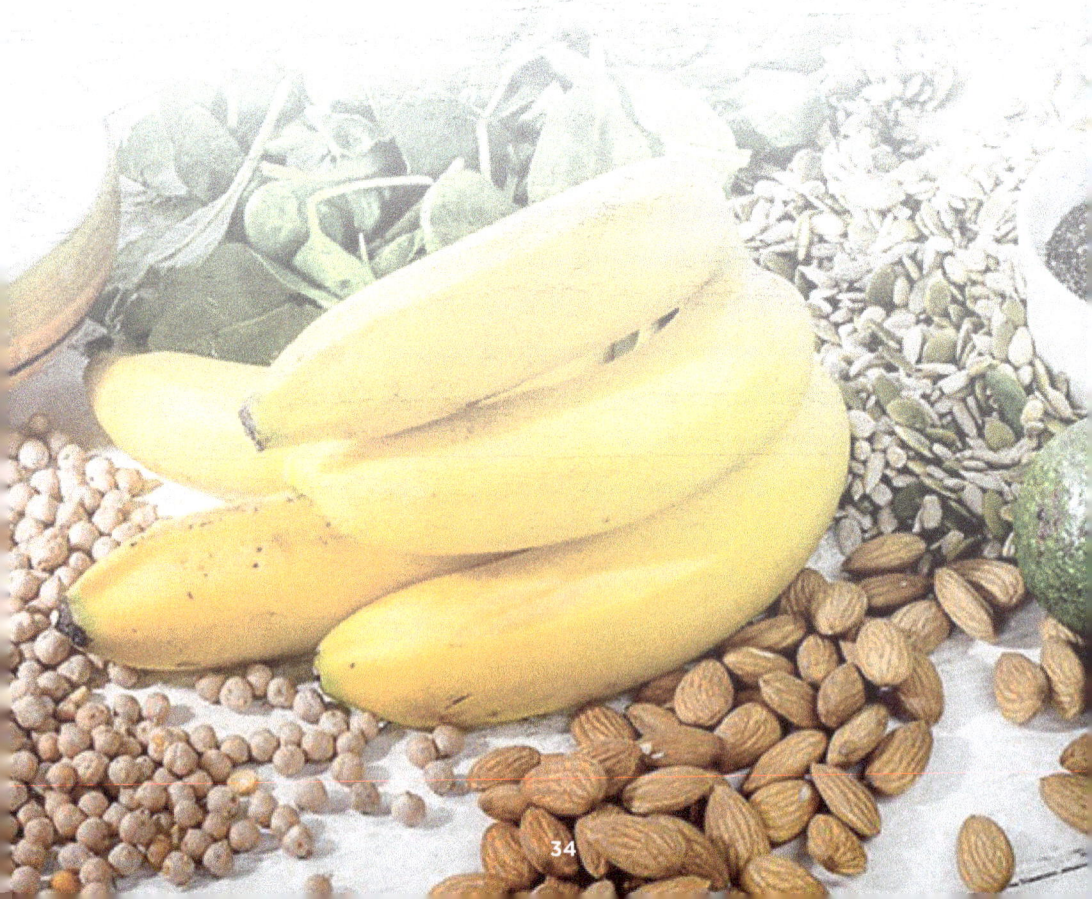

Vitamin D

Vitamin D is another important vitamin that helps the immune system to function properly. It also helps our bodies regulate calcium and phosphorus absorption. This vitamin can be produced in our bodies naturally when we are exposed to sunlight. But most people don't get enough sunlight these days and are generally vitamin D deficient which compromises the immune response to disease.

The best form of vitamin D is cholecalciferol. It is also called vitamin D–3.

Dosage

As a preventive measure when you feel that you are at risk of getting cold or flu or when you start experiencing symptoms, take 400 IU of vitamin D–3 every 3 hours through the day. Don't exceed 2000 IU per day for more than 10 days in a row. Decrease the dosage by 20%–50% and keep taking every 3 hours for at least another 3 to 5 days when you feel that you have recovered.

If you can't get vitamin D–3 in tablet form, you can get it produced in your skin naturally by going out in the sun for 10 to 25 minutes at least 3 times a week. The best time is between 10 am and 3 pm. Make sure you don't get sunburned.

Natural sources of vitamin D

You can also take the natural foods listed below that are quite high in this vitamin:

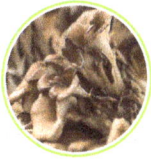

Maitake mushrooms (exposed to ultraviolet light when growing)
1 cup 750 IU

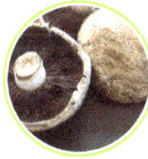

Portobello mushrooms
1 cup – 625 IU

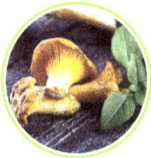

Chanterelle mushrooms (raw)
1 cup – 114 IU

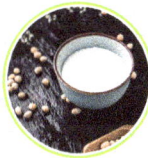

Soy milk (fortified with vitamin D)
1 cup – 120 IU

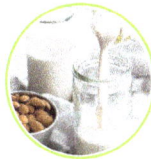

Almond milk (fortified with vitamin D)
1 cup – 100 IU

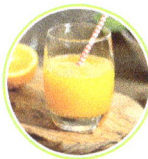

Orange juice (fortified with vitamin D)
1 cup – 100 IU

Zinc

Zinc is a vital mineral that is present in every cell of the body. It plays an important part in protein production, DNA synthesis, cell growth and division along with many other bodily functions.

Zinc boosts the immune system by helping immune cells function and signal properly.

Zinc deficiency can lead to weaker immune system response, which will make it much easier for a cold– or flu–related infection to multiply in the body.

Supplementing with zinc is a proven way to strengthen the immune system, which can help fight off any cold– or flu–related disease in a short time. In one study zinc was found to help shorten the duration of cold symptoms by up to 40%.

Directions

For best results zinc should be taken in small doses throughout the day from morning to night.

Most easily absorbed forms of zinc are: zinc picolinate, zinc citrate and zinc acetate.

When you believe you are at risk of getting cold or flu or when you already have symptoms, take 20 mg of zinc picolinate, citrate or acetate every 3 hours from early morning until 7 pm every day. Take 10 mg to 15 mg every 4–5 hours for another 3 to 5 days after symptoms disappear.

You can mix different forms of zinc; make sure you don't exceed 20 mg of zinc in every 3 hours to avoid overdosing.

Natural sources of zinc

You can also get considerable amounts of zinc from the natural foods listed below if you are unable to get the tablet or capsule forms:

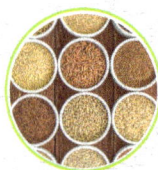

Whole grains: brown rice, quinoa, oats.

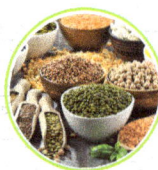

Legumes: black beans, kidney beans, lentils, chickpeas

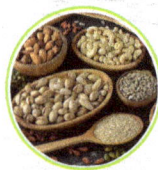

Nuts and seeds: hemp seeds, cashews, pumpkin seeds.

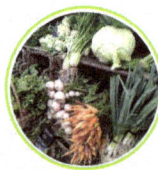

Some vegetables: kale, peas, asparagus, beet greens, mushrooms.

Selenium

Selenium is another powerful mineral which helps the body fight free radicals and protects the cells from oxidative stress. It has a host of benefits which include improving cognitive function, helping bodies stay fertile, keeping the heart healthy and preventing heart disease, preventing mental decline, enabling proper thyroid functioning and most importantly it boosts the immune system which helps the body effectively fight cold– and flu–related infections. Scientists at the University of North Carolina found that viruses can mutate into more harmful forms when bodies are deficient in selenium.

Directions

Take 50 mcg of selenium in tablet form every 3 hours through the day from 7 am until 7 pm when you think you are at risk with no symptoms or when you already have the first symptoms of cold of flu.

Reduce dosage by 50% and take 25 mcg of selenium every 3 hours for another 3–5 days when you recover.

Natural sources of selenium

If you can't get selenium supplements in tablet form, you can always get adequate levels of this important nutrient by consuming the foods listed below that are naturally high in this mineral:

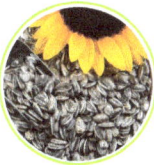

Sunflower seeds
49 mcg per 100g

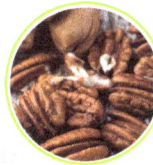

Pecan nuts
12 mcg per 100g

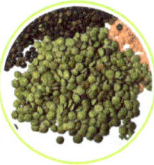

Green or brown lentils
40 mcg per 100g

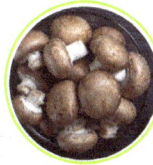

Mushrooms
12 mcg per 100g

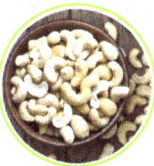

Cashew nuts
34 mcg per 100g

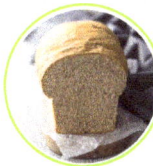

Wholemeal bread
11 mcg per 100g

Copper

Copper is an essential trace mineral that our bodies need for proper functioning of nerve cells, making red blood cells, absorption of iron, forming collagen and production of energy. Copper is present in all tissues and plays an important role in maintaining a healthy immune system. A pioneering researcher on copper, Dr. Bill Keevil, has found that copper is capable of killing superbugs and a type of virus known as coronavirus that is responsible for causing cold–like respiratory disease which could lead to severe cases of pneumonia. Other researchers have also found copper to be effective against some flu viruses which make this trace mineral a very important part of our cold– and flu–fighting arsenal.

Dosage

Take 150 mcg every 3 hours from 7 am till 7 pm when you think you are at risk of getting or when you are already experiencing cold or flu–related symptoms. Take about 75 mcg of copper for another 3–5 days after all symptoms are gone.

Natural sources of copper

If you are unable to obtain copper as a supplement in tablet form, you can include in your diet the foods listed below, which are naturally high in this mineral:

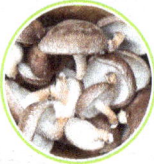

Shiitake Mushrooms approximately four dried mushrooms 89% RDI

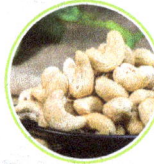

Cashews – 1 ounce (28 grams) 67% RDI

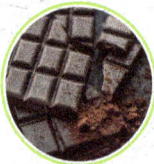

Dark chocolate(70 85% cocoa solids, 25 grams) 50% RDI

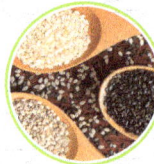

Sesame seeds 1 tablespoon (9 grams) 44% RDI

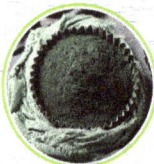

Spirulina 1 tablespoon (7 grams) 44% RDI

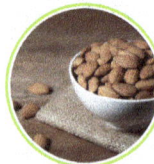

Almonds 1 ounce (28 grams)33% RDI

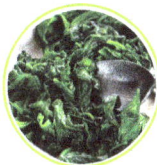

Spinach (Cooked)
1 cup (180 grams)
33% RDI

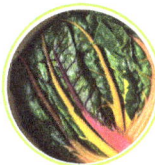

Swiss chard
1cup (173 grams)
33% of the RDI

Where to buy vitamins and supplements

You can buy good quality vitamins in tablets or capsules in local pharmacies, health stores or online

Importance of taking higher doses of nutrients, minerals and vitamins as preventative measure and during the illness

To prevent getting sick or to speed up the recovery process, be sure to take all vitamins and minerals described above in smaller recommended doses every 3–4 hours throughout the day, from 7–8 am until 6–7 pm. This ensures that the immune system has the necessary resources to constantly fight the disease.

Warnings about high doses of vitamins

Don't take Vitamins A, C, D–3, zinc and selenium if you are taking Wellness Formula as it already contains high amounts of these vitamins.

Never take more than 100% of recommended daily intake of any vitamin or mineral for more than 7–9 days in row as it places extra stress on your body.

Always consult your doctor before taking extra vitamins or minerals if you are pregnant or breastfeeding, to ensure you don't have any pre–existing medical conditions and to check that you don't have an allergic or adverse reaction to the vitamins and minerals you intend to take.

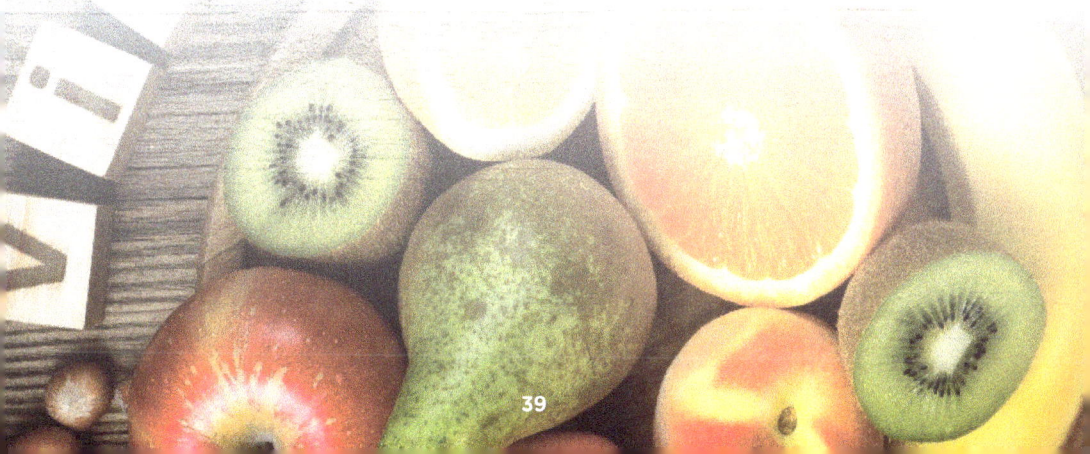

WEAPON 11

TAKE B VITAMINS

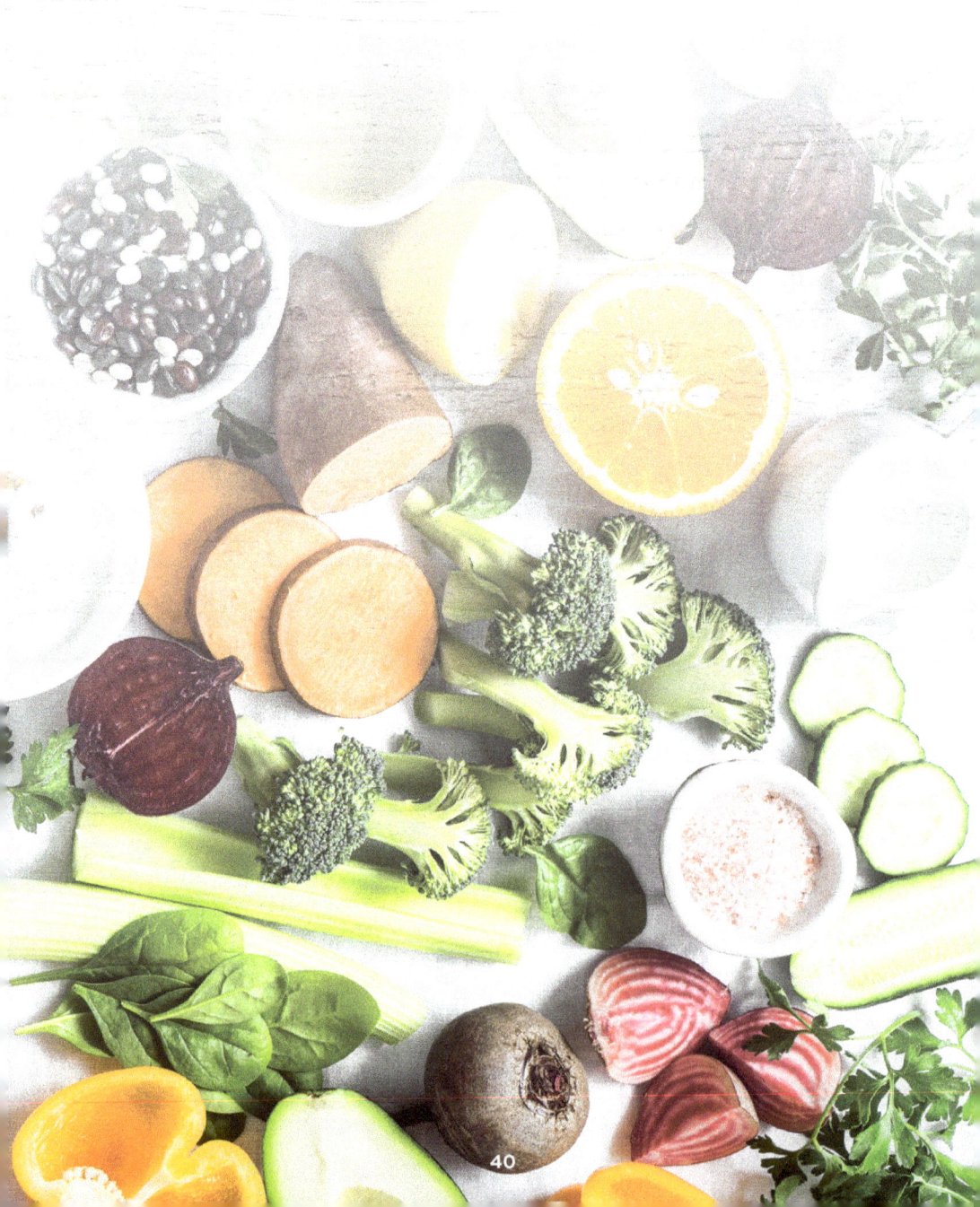

Taking B vitamins while fighting cold or flu is another very important step as deficiency in any vitamin from this group will slow the recovery process considerably. Our bodies need them to function properly.

Some benefits of taking B vitamins include the following: energy production, brain function, cardiovascular health, good digestion, proper nerve function, hormones and cholesterol production, growth of red blood cells and proper immune system function.

Directions

For best results and absorption, B vitamins should be taken in three groups through the day and separately from other vitamins and supplements, at least 1 hour after taking other supplements and vitamins:

First Group - 8:30 am

Take 25 mg of vitamin B–1 (thiamine), 15mg of vitamin B–2 (riboflavin) and 25 mg of vitamin B–3 (niacin);

Second Group - 12 pm

Take 7.5 mg of vitamin B6 in P–5–P form (pyridoxal–5–phosphate) or 15 mg of vitamin B–6 in pyridoxine HCl form together with 200 mcg of vitamin B–7 (biotin), 200 mcg of vitamin B–9 (folate) as calcium folinate (folinic acid) and 50 mg to 100 mg of vitamin B–5 (pantothenic acid).

Third Group - 3:30 pm

Take 25 mg of vitamin B–1 (thiamine), 25 mg to 50 mg of vitamin B–3 (niacin) and 500 mcg of vitamin B–12 as methylcobalamin or 50 mcg of vitamin B–12 as cyanocobalamin.

B vitamins can be taken as general well–being support even when you are not sick. They will provide energy throughout the day and lift your mood. Don't take them every day as you may develop a tolerance. For best results they should be taken in the above–described combinations and dosages every second day. You can also take them for 2–3 days in a row and then stop for another 2–3 days and then repeat the cycle. I prefer to take them on Mondays, Thursdays and Saturdays almost every week.

Where to get good quality B vitamins

You can get good B vitamin supplements online, at your local retail stores and pharmacies.

Natural sources of B vitamins

You can consume the natural foods listed below if you can't get these vitamins as supplements. These foods are naturally rich in B vitamins:

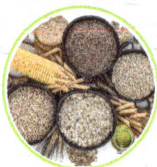

Vitamin B1
Whole grains – wholemeal bread, oats, brown rice and wholewheat pasta; yeast extract – Vegemite or Marmite, nutritional yeast; acorn squash; hazelnuts; pulses – peas, beans and lentils; corn; sesame and sunflower seeds; tahini; brazil nuts, pecan nuts.

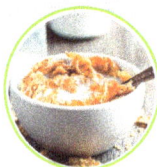

Vitamin B2
Nutritional yeast, yeast extract – Marmite or Vegemite, fortified soy milk, wild rice, snow peas, muesli, mushrooms, fortified vegan breakfast cereals, almonds, avocados, quinoa.

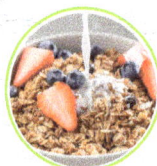

Vitamin B3
Yeast extract – Marmite or Vegemite, nutritional yeast, wild rice, brown rice, quinoa, peanuts, muesli, fortified vegan breakfast cereals, acorn squash, wholewheat pasta, corn.

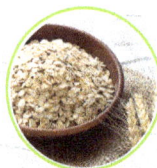

Vitamin B5
Oatmeal and rolled oats, fortified vegan breakfast cereals, nutritional yeast, chestnuts, sweet potatoes, snow peas, avocados, oranges, acorn squash, mushrooms, baked potatoes, plantains, corn, pecan nuts.

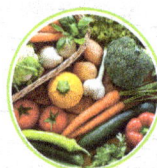

Vitamin B6
Tomatoes, acorn squash, avocados, Brussels sprouts, bananas, fortified vegan breakfast cereals, spring greens, sunflower seeds, chestnuts, corn, wheat germ, quinoa, walnuts, pistachios, whole wheat spaghetti, muesli, hazelnuts, oranges, tahini, sesame seeds, nutritional yeast.

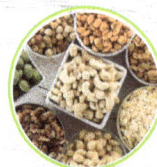

Vitamin B7
Oatmeal or rolled oats, muesli, wheat germ, mushrooms, hazelnuts, almonds, peanuts and peanut butter, walnuts, pistachios, pecans, nutritional yeast, avocados, sunflower and sesame seeds, tahini, tempeh, fortified breakfast cereals.

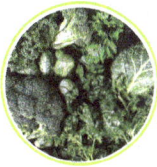

Vitamin B9

Tofu, fortified breakfast cereal, cherry tomatoes, acorn squash, oranges, green vegetables – asparagus, kale, pak choi, broccoli, rocket, spinach, Brussels sprouts, lettuce, peas, sweetcorn, white cabbage, edamame, hazelnuts, tempeh, soy milk, yeast extract – Marmite or Vegemite, red pepper, nutritional yeast, lentils, beetroot, wheat germ, muesli.

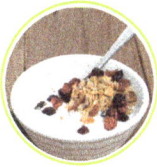

Vitamin B12

Nutritional yeast fortified with B12, B12–fortified plant–based butter, B12–fortified dairy–free yoghurts and desserts, B12–fortified breakfast cereals, B12–fortified plant milks.

Warnings

As with any other new supplements, consult your doctor before taking new vitamins if you are pregnant or breastfeeding, if you have pre–existing medical conditions and to determine if you are allergic to some new substances.

Always read labels carefully and never overdose on a vitamin as it can harm your health.

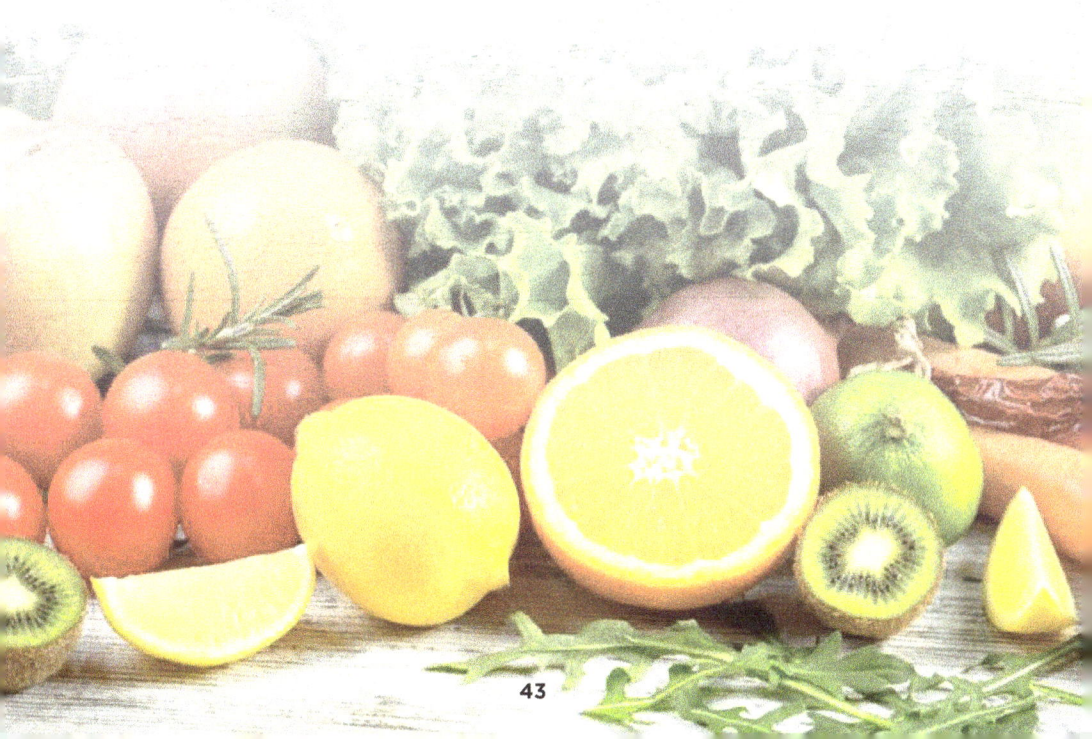

TAKE RAW GINGER, TURMERIC AND CAYENNE PEPPER

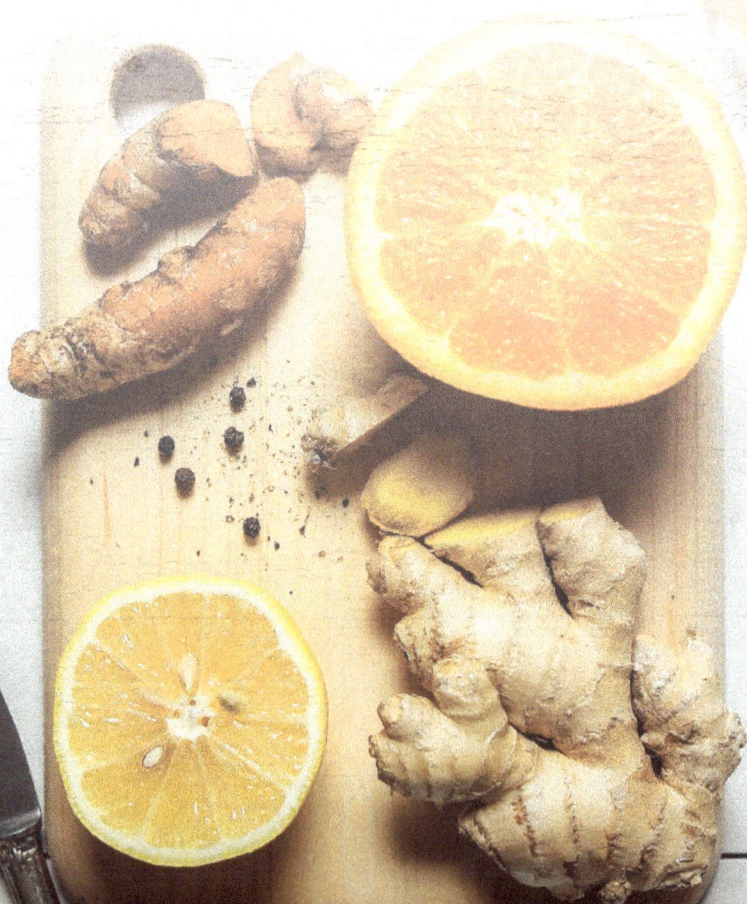

Ginger, turmeric and cayenne pepper are among the healthiest spices that you can add to your diet. Each offers numerous health benefits.

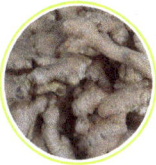

Some benefits of taking ginger include the following: reduction of inflammation, antioxidant activity, protection against toxins and various pathogens, improvement in brain function, reduction in period pain for women, improved digestion, help with morning sickness, lowering of blood sugar levels, improvement in immune system response. In one study ginger was found to enhance the virus killing ability of the immune system, reduce sore throat symptoms and shorten overall duration of cold and flu symptoms.

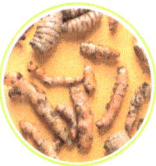

Some benefits of taking turmeric include: reduces inflammation, enhances brain–derived neurotrophic factor which leads to improved brain function, better memory and a lower risk of brain diseases, powerful antioxidant action, proven anti–depressant, reduces symptoms of arthritis, stronger immune system response. Similar to ginger, turmeric also has the ability to effectively kill some viruses including cold and flu–related ones.

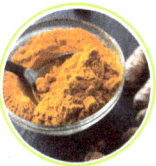

Cayenne pepper is a true miracle plant with many great health benefits. Some amazing benefits include: increases metabolism, detoxifies the body, has positive effect on digestive system, possesses anti–bacterial, anti–viral and anti–fungal properties. Cayenne pepper is also a very effective remedy against cold and flu. It can break up, mobilize and remove mucus from the body; it can also raise the body's temperature which helps kill viral and bacterial infections, and it contains vitamin C which strengthens the immune system. The above benefits make cayenne pepper a very effective addition to your cold and flu–fighting arsenal. To more thoroughly understand the beneficial effects of cayenne pepper, I highly recommend to read Left for Dead by Richard Quinn.

How to take ginger, turmeric and cayenne pepper

Cayenne pepper can be taken in raw, capsule or powder forms. If taking it raw, bite off a tiny 1–3 mm piece and chew thoroughly. If you find taking it raw is too hot and overwhelming, you can add a small pinch of cayenne pepper powder to a quarter or half glass of warm water and drink it.

Ginger and Turmeric can also be taken in raw, capsule or powder forms.

If taking them raw cut approximately two to three square centimetres of raw ginger and raw turmeric, peel well with a sharp knife or a potato peeler and chew a small 1–3 square millimetres piece of each – ginger and turmeric – every couple of hours throughout the day while you are experiencing cold or flu–related symptoms. Make sure to chew them thoroughly for at least 30 seconds or more to enhance digestion.

Curcumin is a bioactive compound which is responsible for most of the health benefits of turmeric. For better absorption, turmeric and curcumin should be taken with some black pepper or black pepper extract as piperine in black pepper increases the absorption of curcumin by up to 2000%.

Apart from making the immune system stronger and speeding up your cold and flu recovery times, ginger, turmeric and cayenne pepper will enhance the overall feeling of well–being and clarity of mind.

Warnings

Don't take too much raw ginger, turmeric or cayenne pepper! Experiment with your ideal portion size until you find what works for you without negative side effects. If you take too much of either, you may experience a mild headache that could last for up to an hour or two as these spices contain many medicinal compounds that may overwhelm the brain.

Start taking them in very small doses at first and increase gradually according to your personal reaction. Usually it is recommended to take a slightly smaller piece of turmeric and slightly bigger piece of ginger.

Turmeric can also make your teeth look yellow. It is only temporary and can be removed with a toothbrush. You can chew turmeric with back teeth to avoid staining the front ones.

Also be careful with cayenne pepper. Start with very small doses and see how your body reacts. Increase dosage very gradually. Cayenne pepper can cause heartburn–like symptoms and other digestive discomforts if you are not used to it.

To avoid digestive discomfort, don't take ginger, turmeric and cayenne pepper on an empty stomach and consume food right after taking them.

Where to get them

Ginger, turmeric and cayenne pepper can be found in many local grocery stores or online.

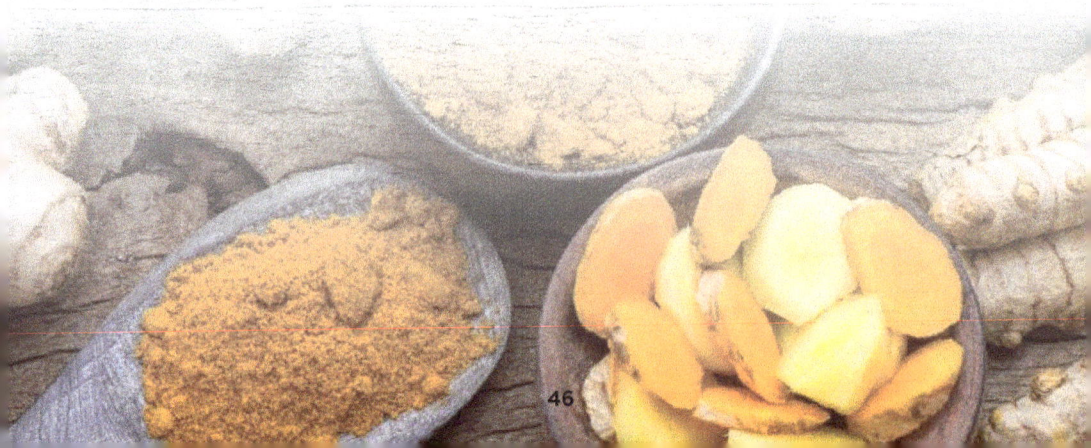

WEAPON 13

TAKE HORSERADISH AND GARLIC

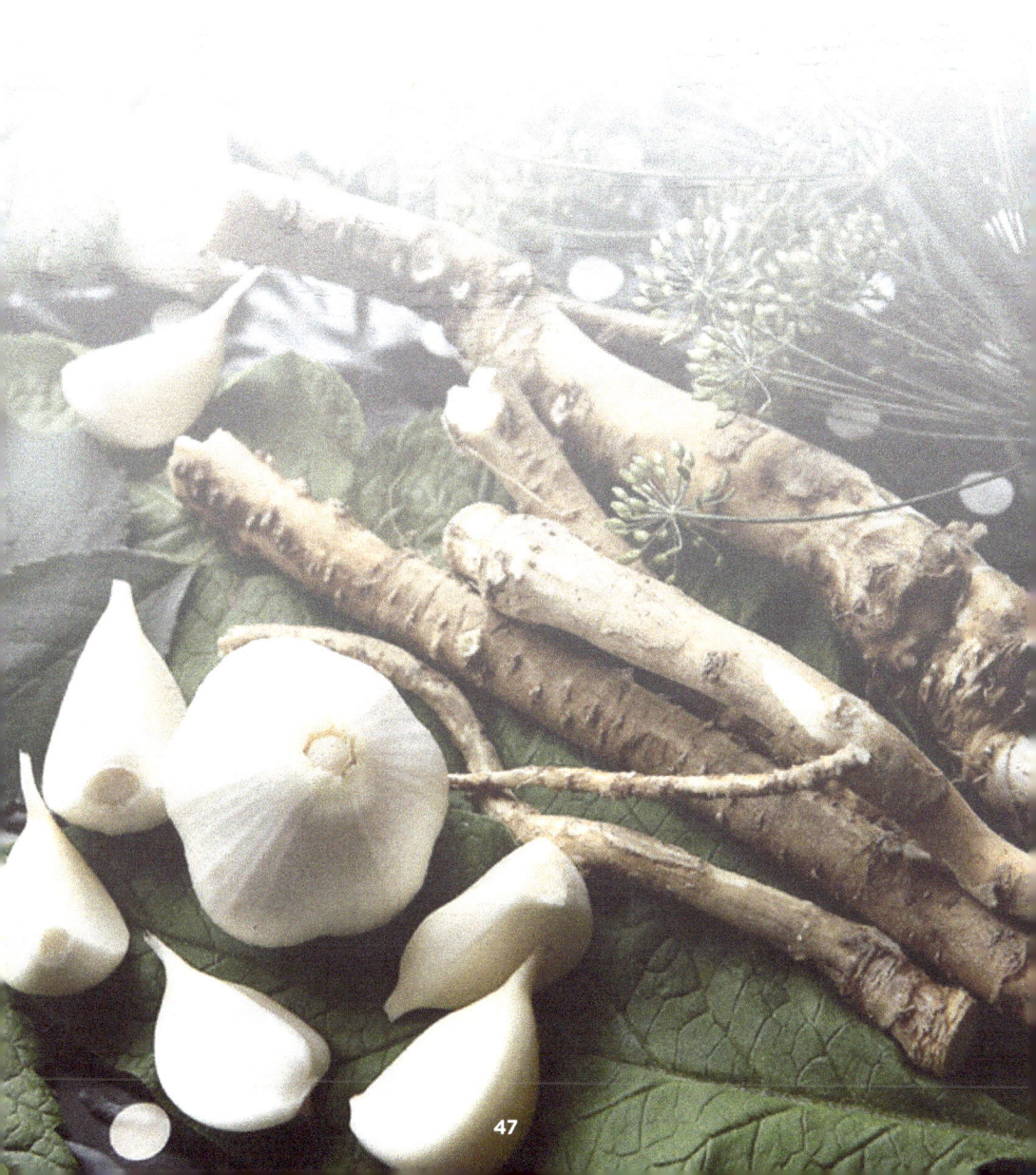

Combining horseradish and garlic is yet another effective way to prevent or speed up recovery from cold or flu.

Some benefits of taking horseradish include that it acts as an antibacterial agent, pain and inflammation relief, helps digestion, improves metabolism, regulates blood pressure, treats sinus and urinary tract infections, and strengthens the immune system.

Horseradish can be very effective in your disease–fighting arsenal as it is a proven remedy that can effectively fight cold and flu by shortening the duration and relieving the symptoms of those maladies. In some studies horseradish was found to increase immune system response by up to 4000 times and to effectively treat and relieve the symptoms of sinus and upper respiratory tract infections.

Garlic is another miracle plant with a host of health benefits. It has been used for centuries to effectively treat various health conditions. It can also be an effective addition to your diet when you are trying to recover from cold or flu.

Some benefits of taking garlic: can reduce blood pressure, help detoxify the body of heavy metals, act as a potent antioxidant and lower cholesterol. Garlic possesses antibiotic properties, is beneficial for heart and liver health, and strengthens the immune system. Through different studies, garlic showed potential to reduce the severity of symptoms, duration and frequency of cold and flu.

Directions

Horseradish

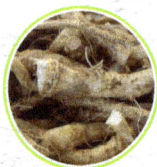

If you are lucky you may be able to buy fresh, raw horseradish root at your local fruit shop, supermarket or online. This is the best form to take. Peel approximately 5 mm to 1 cm piece and bite 1–3 mm and chew thoroughly for at least 30 seconds.

If you can't find raw horseradish root, you can always take a small amount of hot wasabi or horseradish paste instead. For best results wasabi or horseradish paste should be very hot and spicy—not mild—and must contain at least 50% – 90% of horseradish.

Garlic

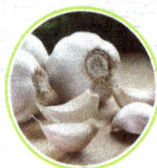

Best taken in the raw form. Peel one clove of garlic and chew a 2–3 mm piece thoroughly.

If you feel that horseradish and garlic are too hot or too spicy to take on their own, you can add them to salads, eat them with a piece of bread or mix them with other food.

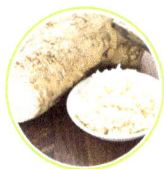

Horseradish and garlic should be taken every 3–4 hours while experiencing symptoms of cold or flu. You can take horseradish and garlic with ginger, turmeric and cayenne pepper or you can take them an hour or longer apart.

Warnings

Horseradish and garlic are quite spicy and may cause digestive heartburn–like discomfort if you are not used to them. Start with small doses and gradually increase the portion sizes as your body adapts.

To avoid digestive discomfort, don't take horseradish and garlic on an empty stomach and eat food right after taking them.

Garlic will make your breath smell like garlic. To reduce this side–effect, rinse your mouth, take breath freshening lozenges or brush your teeth lightly after taking garlic.

If you can't tolerate taking raw garlic, horseradish, wasabi or horseradish and garlic pastes, you can instead take them as a supplement in tablet or capsule forms.

Where to obtain horseradish and garlic

You can buy garlic and horseradish in raw, paste and supplement forms online or in local supermarkets, health food stores and pharmacies.

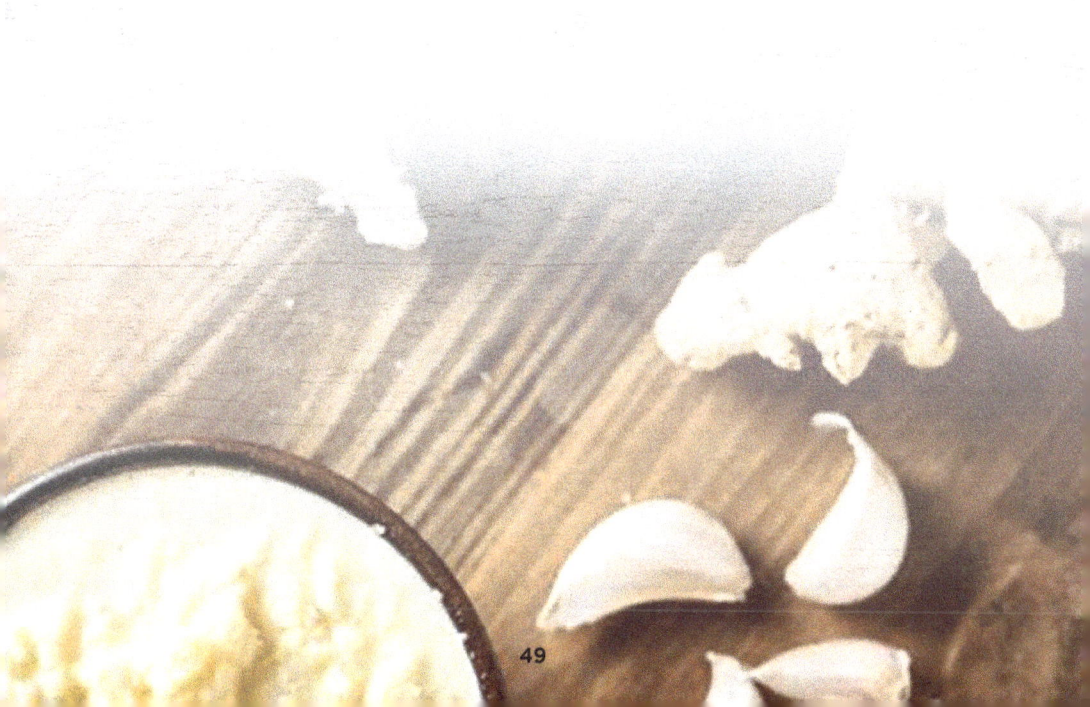

WEAPON 14

TAKE ROSEHIPS, HIBISCUS, ECHINACEA AND ELDERBERRY

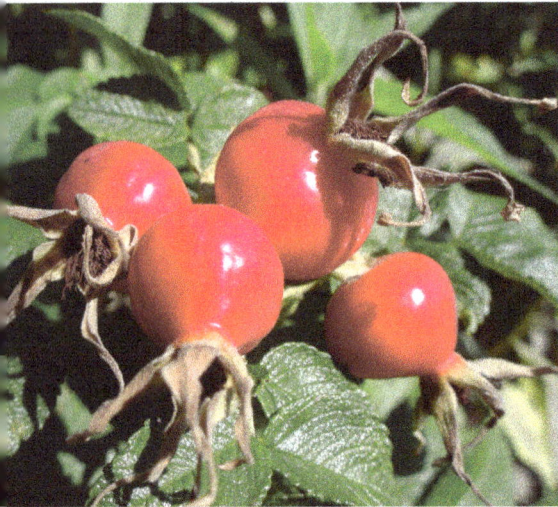

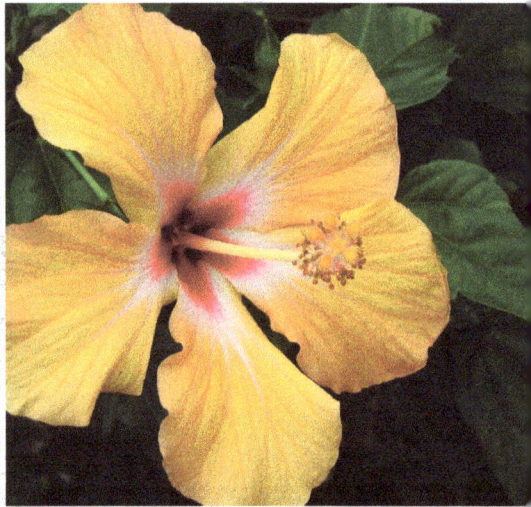

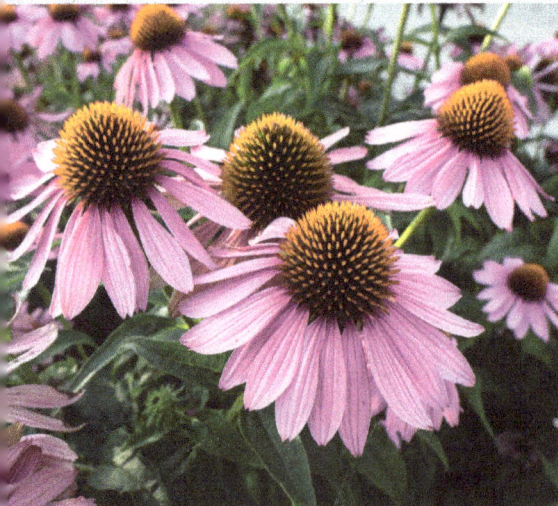

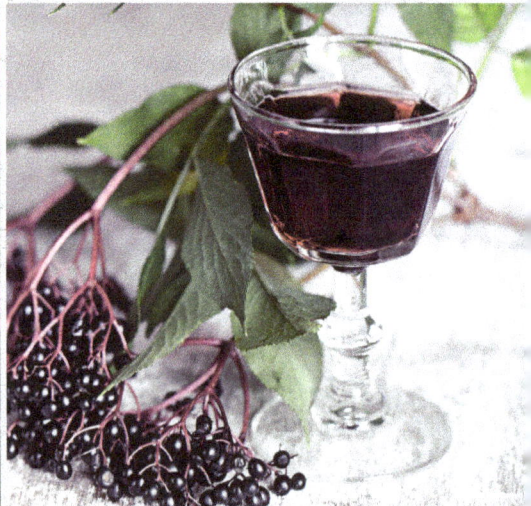

Rosehips, hibiscus, echinacea and elderberry are all capable of boosting the immune system. When used together, their combined immune system support is much stronger and can help reduce the symptoms and fight off cold or flu–related illnesses.

Benefits

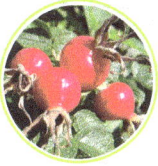

Rosehips
May be beneficial against heart disease, type 2 diabetes; can slow the aging process of the skin; can reduce inflammation and pain symptoms; high antioxidant activity; high in vitamin C which supports the immune system.

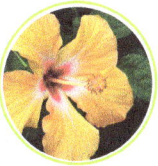

Hibiscus
Has antibacterial properties; can lower cholesterol; may lower blood pressure; has positive effects on our digestive system, heart, kidneys and liver functions; may assist with weight loss; is high in antioxidants; contains high levels of immune boosting vitamin C.

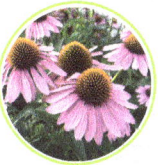

Echinacea
Can help with blood sugar control; may reduce blood pressure and inflammation levels; has antioxidant properties; may increase the number of white blood cells which help the body fight infections.

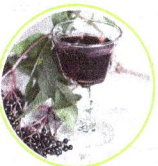

Elderberry
High in free radicals fighting antioxidants; can reduce inflammation; is beneficial for heart health; has antibacterial activity; is high in vitamin C, which can support the immune system. Different studies demonstrate that elderberry can significantly reduce the duration and severity of symptoms of cold– and flu–related diseases.

Directions

For best immune boosting results take them together as a hot drink. Add half to one teaspoon of echinacea, hibiscus, rosehips and elderberries to a cup of boiling water and let it steep for around 5–10 minutes before drinking. Drink this hot beverage at least every 3–4 hours while you are sick or as a preventive measure when you think you are at risk of getting sick.

For even greater immune–boosting effect, it is highly recommended to take extra elderberry extract or syrup in capsule, lozenges or tablet forms.

Organic forms are preferred as they are grown almost without chemicals.

Where to get them

You can get them online or locally in trusted health stores.

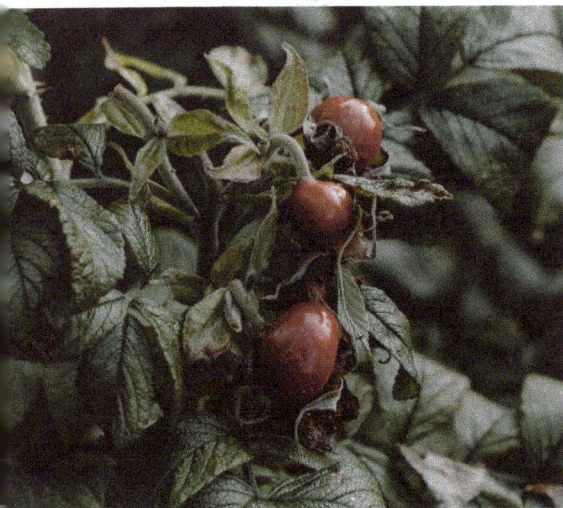

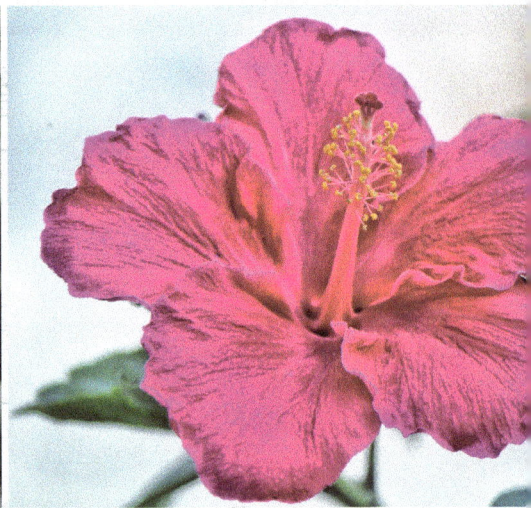

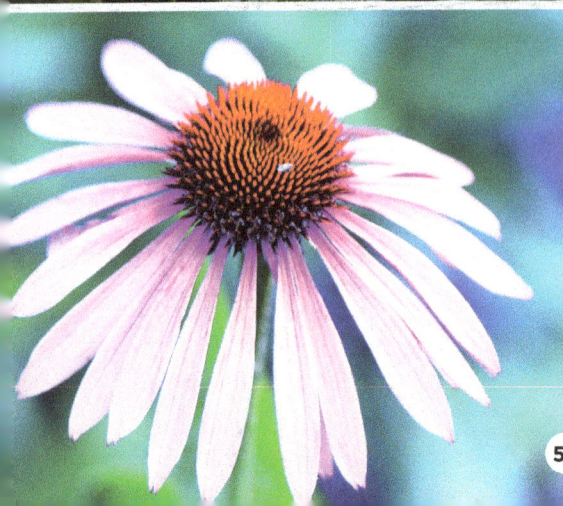

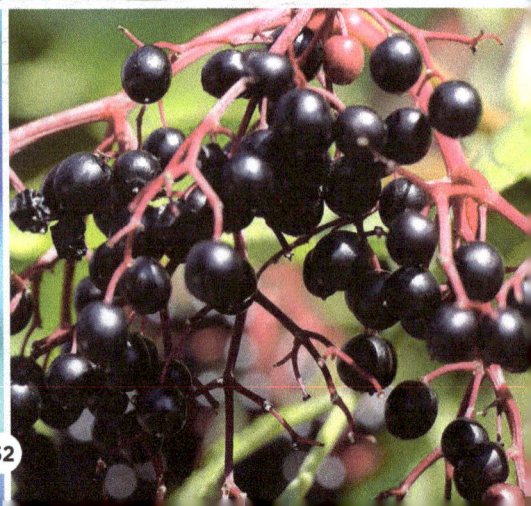

WEAPON 15

DRINK APPLE CIDER VINEGAR WITH CAYENNE PEPPER, CINNAMON AND LEMON JUICE

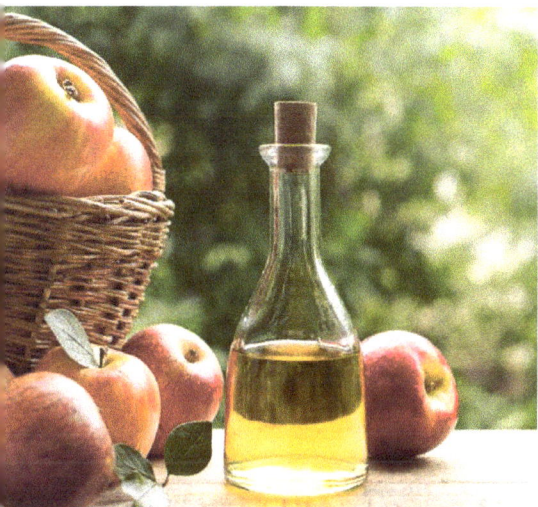

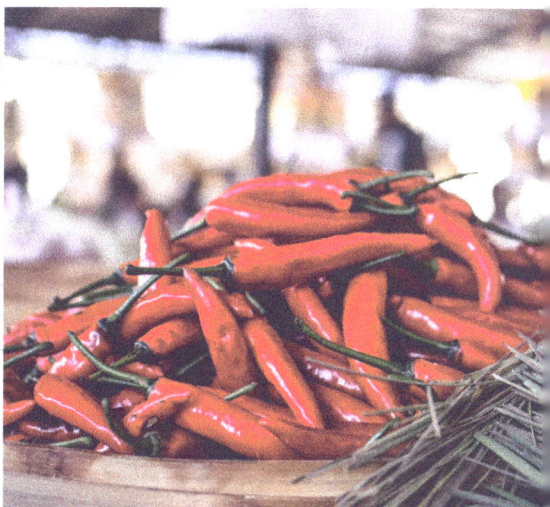

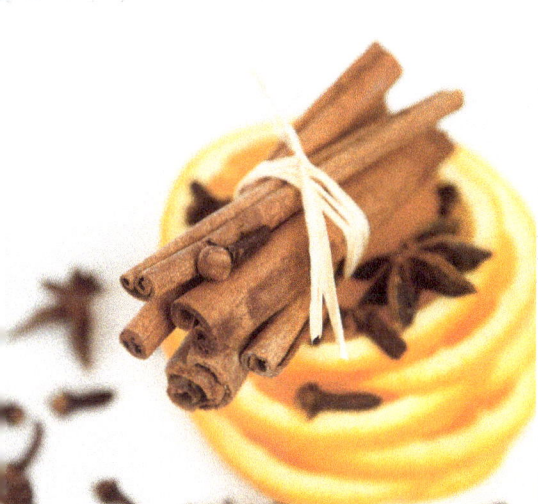

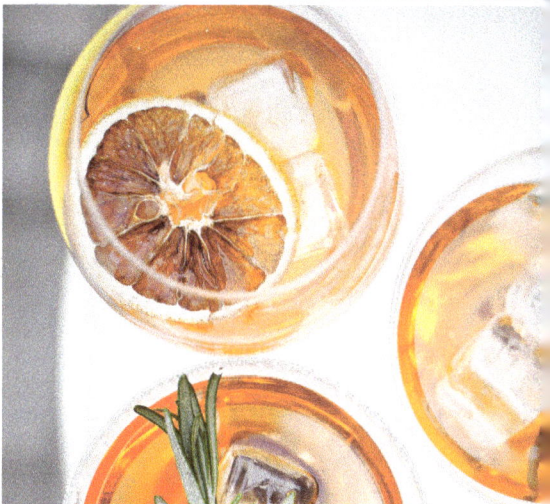

This drink combines four powerful ingredients: apple cider vinegar, cayenne pepper, cinnamon and lemon juice which are quite effective at treating and relieving cold and flu symptoms.

Benefits

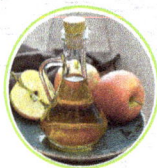

Apple cider vinegar
Can alkalize the body and help dissolve the mucus in the respiratory system, which will help you feel better and speed up the recovery process.

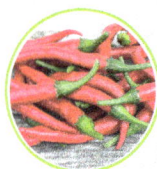

Cayenne Pepper
Please refer to chapter "Weapon 12" to read about benefits of cayenne pepper.

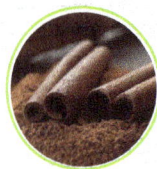

Cinnamon
Lowers blood sugar levels; has antiviral, antibiotic, anti–fungal and anti–bacterial properties; is a potent antioxidant with anti–inflammatory action; beneficial for nervous system and may prevent Alzheimer's disease; beneficial for healthy heart function; can improve insulin sensitivity; is very high in antioxidants that can boost and support the immune system which may help fight off cold and flu naturally. Cinnamon has been used in China and India for centuries to treat the common cold and relieve sore throat.

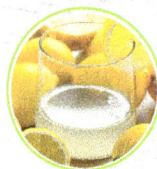

Lemon Juice
Acts as an antioxidant; beneficial for kidneys and liver health; aids digestion; promotes hydration; has pH balancing alkalizing properties; may improve mood; is also rich in immune–system–supporting vitamin C, which makes it effective at fighting cold and flu.

Directions

In a mug of hot water, add one–half to 2 tablespoons of apple cider vinegar, a small pinch of cayenne pepper and cinnamon, along with juice from a quarter to a half of lemon. Mix well. Let it steep for a few minutes and drink slowly while it is still warm.

You can add a little maple syrup or raspberry jam for a sweeter drink.

Apart from supporting the immune system and helping fight off cold or flu, this drink may lift your mood and improve overall clarity of mind and sense of well–being.

Warnings

Don't take too much of any ingredient in this drink as each may cause digestive system discomfort if you are not used to them. Start with very small doses of each ingredient and increase slowly as your body adjusts. Taking some foods before and after this drink may help to avoid digestive discomfort. Don't take vinegar if you have an ulcer. Always consult your doctor before adding new supplements to your diet!

All of the above ingredients can be bought locally in your favorite shops or online.

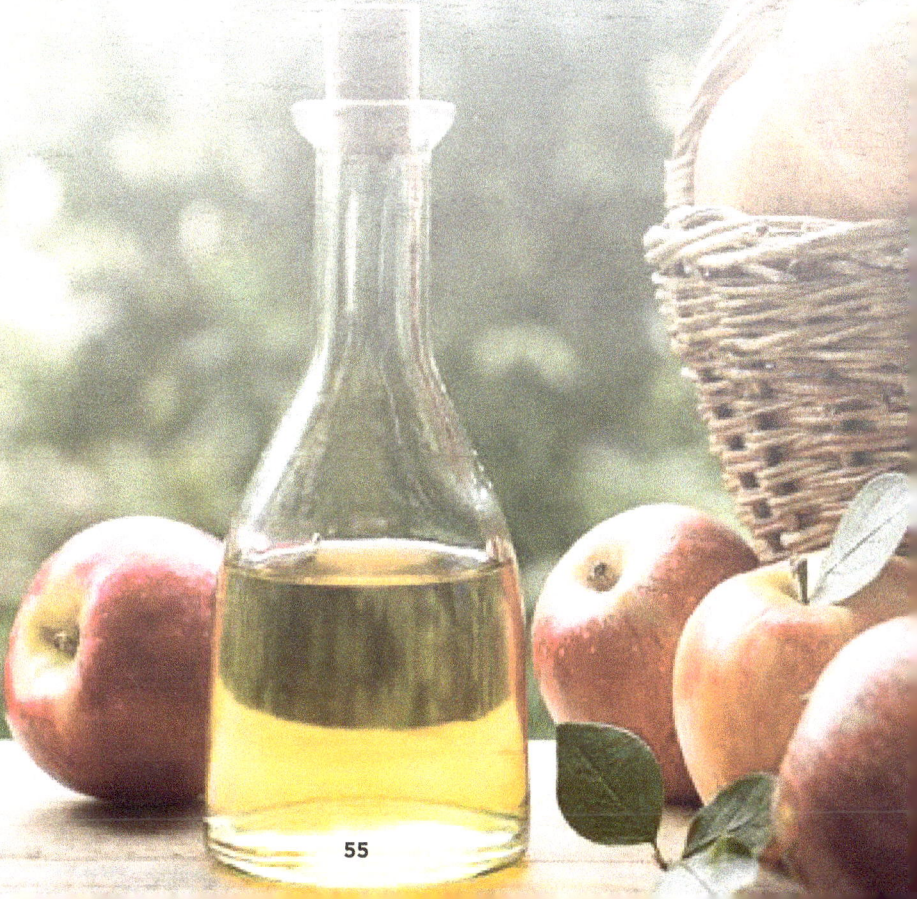

WEAPON 16

TAKE MEDICINAL MUSHROOMS

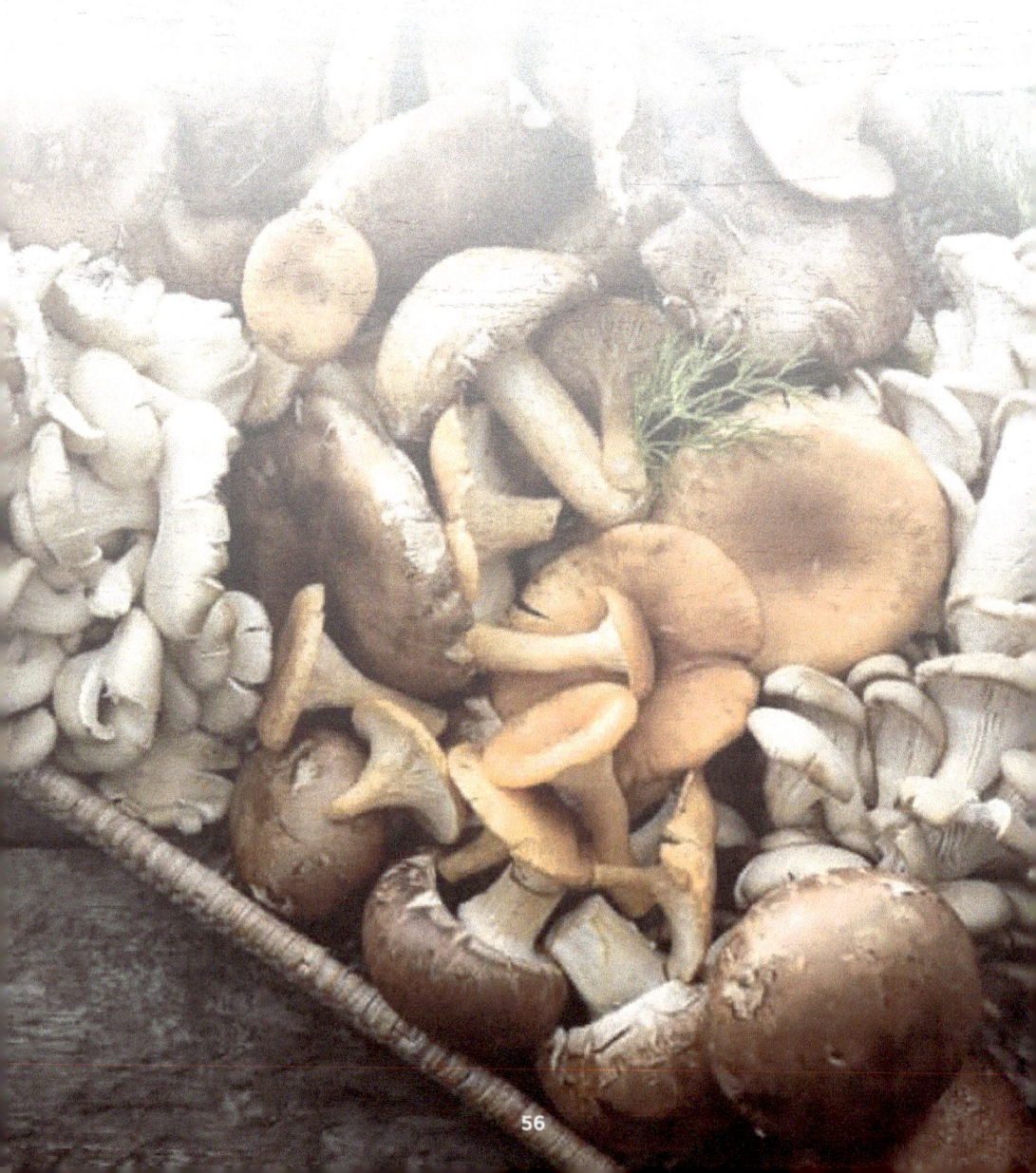

Taking medicinal mushrooms is yet another great way to enhance overall health and strengthen the immune system. The mushrooms described below have been used to treat various ailments for centuries and can have a great positive impact on our ability to fight off cold– and flu–related infections.

Taking medicinal mushrooms offers a multitude of health benefits that go far beyond fighting cold and flu. Listed below are some benefits:

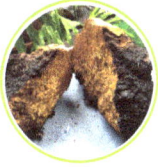

Chaga – anti–oxidant, anti–inflammatory, anti–bacterial, anti–viral and anti–fungal properties; can lower blood pressure, blood sugar and cholesterol levels; may slow aging; may help prevent blood clotting; good for skin, brain, heart, digestive system and liver health; can boost the immune system by stimulating the production of beneficial cytokines, by supporting white blood cells and by serving as a source of beta–glucans and other necessary minerals and micro–nutrients.

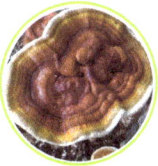

Reishi – anti–oxidant, anti–inflammatory and anti–viral properties; may help with low energy levels and depression; may improve sleep; may lower blood sugar, cholesterol and blood pressure levels; good for brain, prostate, liver, kidneys, digestive system, cardiovascular system and heart health; can boost the immune system due to polysaccharides content and by stimulating white blood cells and the genes within.

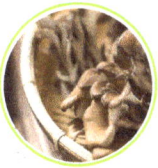

Maitake – anti–oxidant and anti–viral properties; may lower blood sugar, blood pressure and cholesterol levels; may help treat polycystic ovary syndrome; good for digestive system, heart and cardiovascular system health; can support the immune system due to polysaccharides and various other micro–nutrients contents.

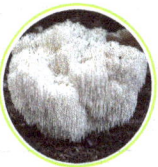

Lions Mane – anti–inflammatory and anti–oxidant properties; can lift mood, improve memory and cognitive abilities; may lower blood sugar levels; may help treat anxiety and depression; may improve sleep quality; may help prevent dementia and Alzheimer's disease; may help regenerate and grow new nerve cells; good for heart, digestive system and brain health; can boost the immune system due to polysaccharides and various other micro–nutrients contents.

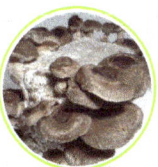

Shiitake – anti–oxidant, anti–inflammatory, anti–viral, anti–microbial and anti–bacterial properties; may lower cholesterol and blood pressure levels; may help prevent anaemia; may prevent auto–immune diseases; good for eyes, hair, skin, brain, prostate, liver, bones, heart, cardiovascular system and digestive system health; can boost the immune system due to polysaccharides, zinc, B group vitamins, iron, vitamin D and various other micronutrients contents.

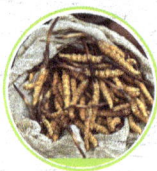

Cordyceps – anti–oxidant and anti–inflammatory properties; may improve athletic performance and elevate energy levels; may help boost libido; may help treat asthma; may lower cholesterol, blood sugar and blood pressure levels; good for brain, liver, kidneys, heart and endocrine system health; can boost the immune system due to polysaccharides and various other micro–nutrients contents.

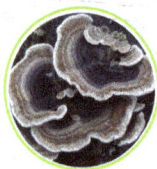

Turkey Tail – antioxidant, anti–inflammatory, antibiotic, antifungal and anti–bacterial properties; may lower blood sugar and blood pressure levels; may help treat human papillomavirus (HPV); may help improve physical performance; good for teeth, bones, liver, heart, cardiovascular system and digestive system health; can boost the immune system due to polysaccharides, PSP and PSK polysaccharopeptides and various other micro–nutrients contents.

How to take medicinal mushrooms

For best immune–boosting results, take the mushrooms described above together as a complex.

I highly recommend starting with Immune Defence mushrooms complex capsules made by a reputable Fungi Perfecti brand. It is one of the best medicinal mushrooms products on the market at the time of writing these lines (September 2020) and it has a proven record that it works to strengthen the immune system and effectively prevent or fight off cold– and flu–related diseases.

Another great medicinal mushrooms complex product is Mushroom Immune Defence by Source Naturals.

I also recommend trying the above described mushrooms one by one — separately — to see how you feel after taking them and how your body responds to each one.

Warnings

Don't take multi mushrooms complex powders, capsules or tablets while taking individual mushrooms supplements and vice versa. Don't take individual mushrooms powders, capsules or tablets while taking multi–mushrooms products as you may overdose on certain mushrooms which can have a negative effect on your health.

As with any new supplements, consult your doctor before adding medicinal mushrooms to your diet, especially if you are pregnant or breastfeeding.

Also before taking, ensure you don't have pre–existing medical conditions, that you are not allergic and don't have adverse reactions to a medicinal mushroom.

While they are safe for most people, they may be harmful to your health if you have a pre–existing medical condition or if you are allergic to certain substances.

Carefully read the labels to determine permitted safe dosages and never overdose when taking the medicinal mushrooms described in this chapter.

Where to purchase

You can buy medicinal mushrooms powders, capsules or tablets in most local health stores, some pharmacies or online.

Highly recommended multiple mushrooms products:

Hots Defense MyCommunity 17 Mushrooms Complex by Fungi Perfecti

Mushroom Immune Defence 15 mushrooms complex by Source Naturals

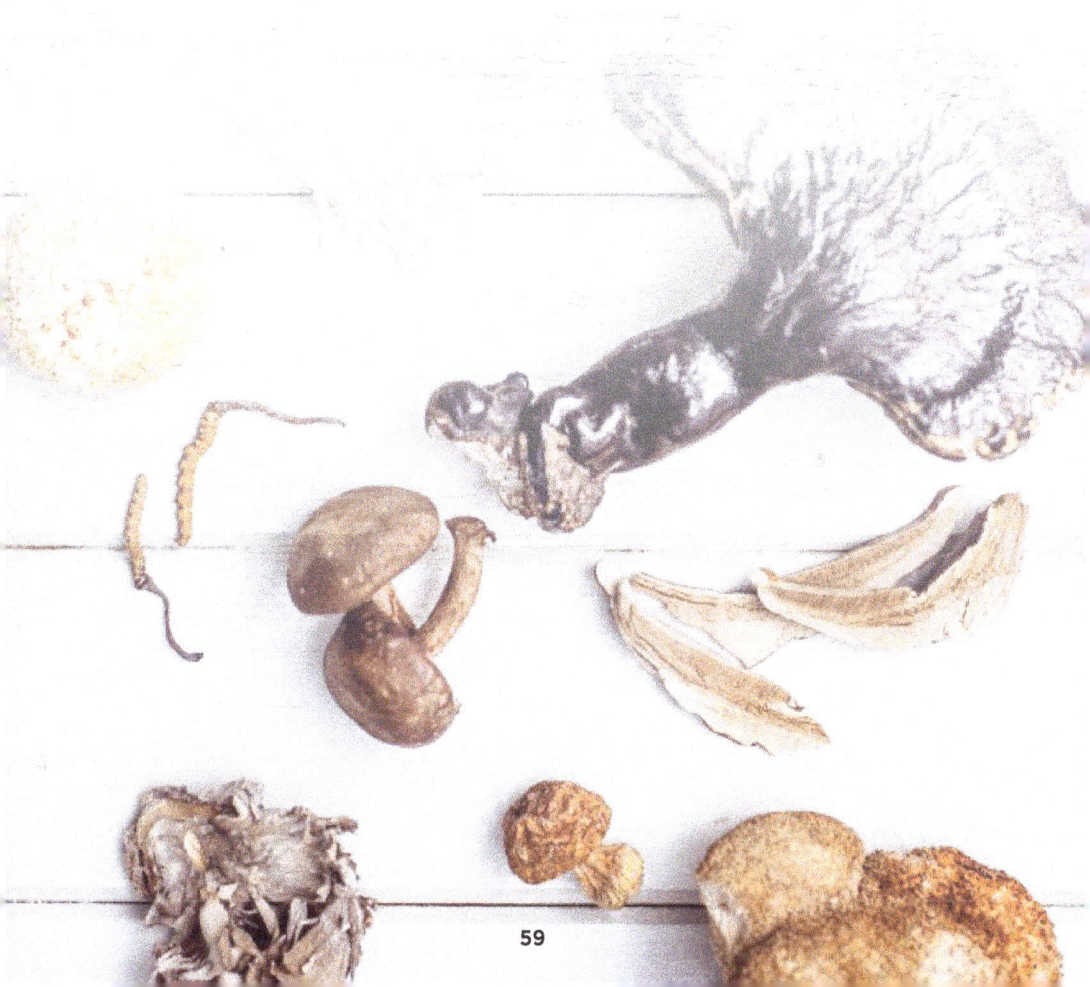

WEAPON 17

TAKE VEGAN PROTEIN, GLUTAMINE AND BCAA SUPPLEMENTS

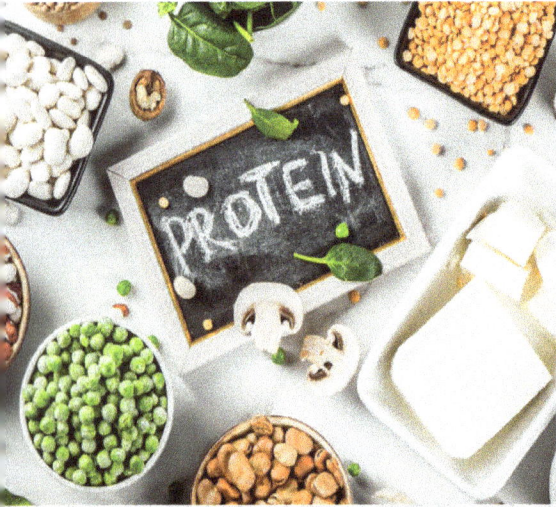

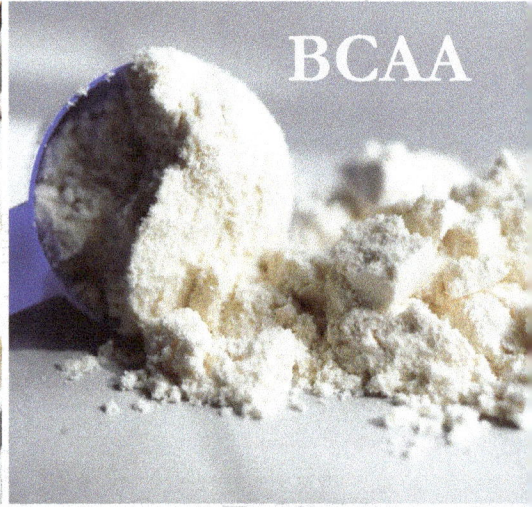

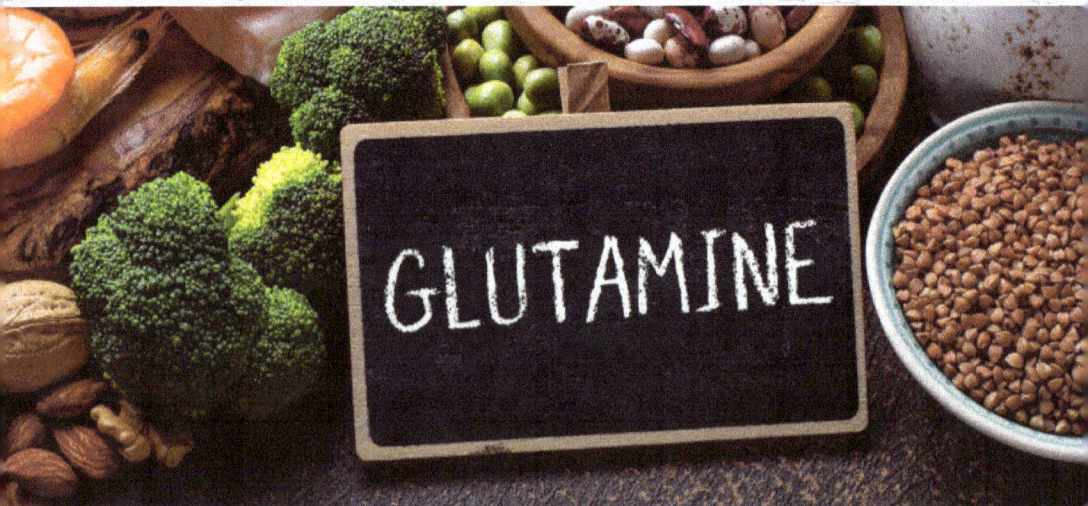

Vegan protein, glutamine and BCAA (Branched–Chain Amino Acids) are effective supplements that can strengthen the immune system and help the body recover from cold– or flu–related infections.

Below are some benefits of adding them to your diet

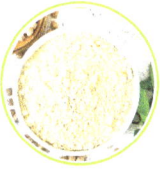

Vegan protein (blends of pea and rice protein) – can boost metabolism; can help you stay stronger and build muscles; good for skin, hair, brain, cardiovascular system and digestive system health; can boost the immune system due to various amino acids contents. Make sure that you get vegan protein with complete amino acids profile. It must contain a mix of pea and rice proteins. Always read the label on protein to ensure it has complete amino acids profile and does not contain artificial ingredients.

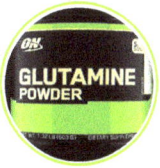

Glutamine – can improve wound healing and post exercise recovery times; can help with anxiety and mood control; can help with ulcers and leaky gut; good for brain and digestive system health; can prevent muscle catabolism; can help control blood sugar level; can boost the immune system as it is a source of fuel for immune cells.

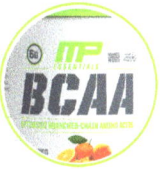

BCAA – Branched–Chain Amino Acids – leucine, isoleucine, valine – provide the body with a source of energy that can improve aerobic and anaerobic performance; can prevent muscle catabolism, decrease muscle soreness, reduce muscle fatigue and increase muscle synthesis after physical activities; may help with fat loss; can help manage liver disease and regulate blood sugar levels; can strengthen and help regenerate the immune system by providing a source of energy to immune cells.

How to take vegan protein, glutamine and BCAA

Mix approximately 15–25 grams of vegan protein in half a cup of cold water; then add 1–3 grams of glutamine and 1–3 grams of BCAA powders and mix until all ingredients are dissolved and form a smoothie–like drink. You can use a protein shaker, NutriBullet or similar blender to speed up the mixing process. Take this drink every 4–5 hours from early morning till about 5 pm while you are experiencing symptoms of cold or flu or as a preventative measure. Even if you are not sick and not at risk of getting sick, this protein and amino acids drink will make you feel stronger and energized. It is also a great mix to use before and after exercise to achieve faster recovery times. To make it sweeter you can add natural sweeteners like maple or agave syrups, berries or fruits.

Warnings

Don't take vegan protein, BCAA and glutamine after 5 pm as they may interfere with sleep. Don't take too much vegan protein, BCAA or glutamine. Read the labels carefully and never exceed recommended dosages.

Consult your doctor before adding new supplements to your diet if you are pregnant, breastfeeding, have pre–existing medical conditions and to make sure you are not allergic to the supplements.

Where to buy vegan protein, BCAA and glutamine

You can buy vegan protein, BCAA and glutamine supplements at local health stores or online.

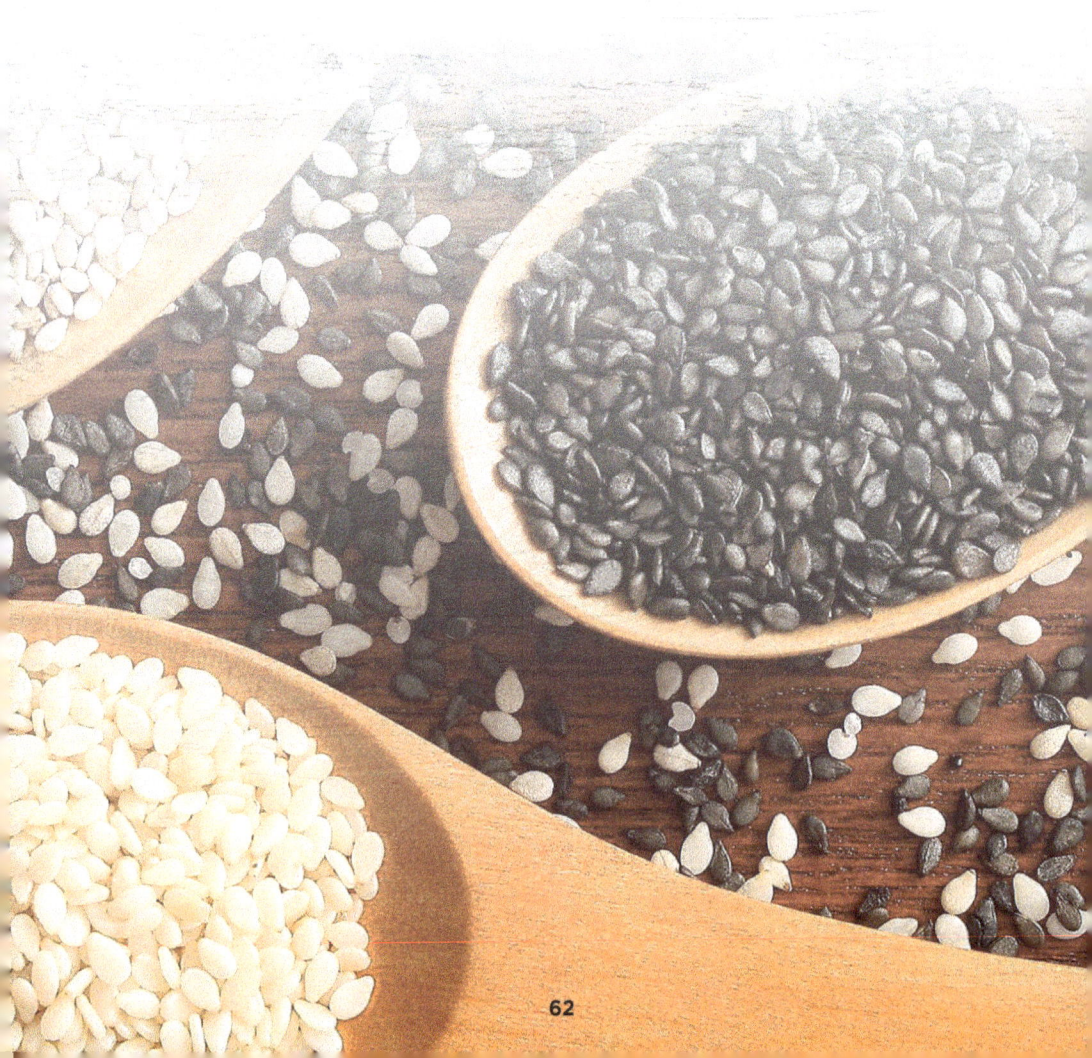

TAKE HEALTHY FATS — BLACK SEED, OREGANO, FLAXSEED AND MEDIUM CHAIN TRIGLYCERIDES (MCT) OILS

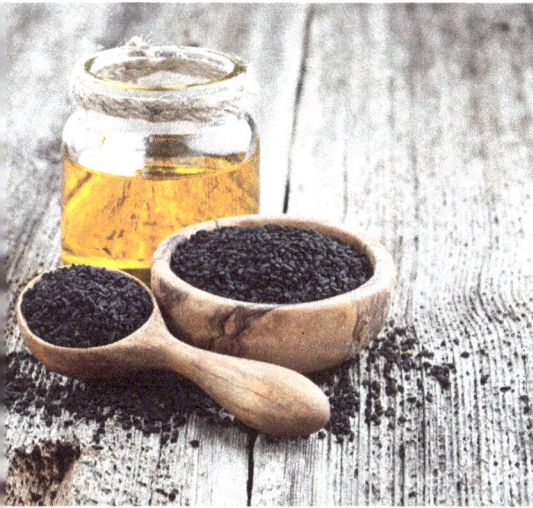

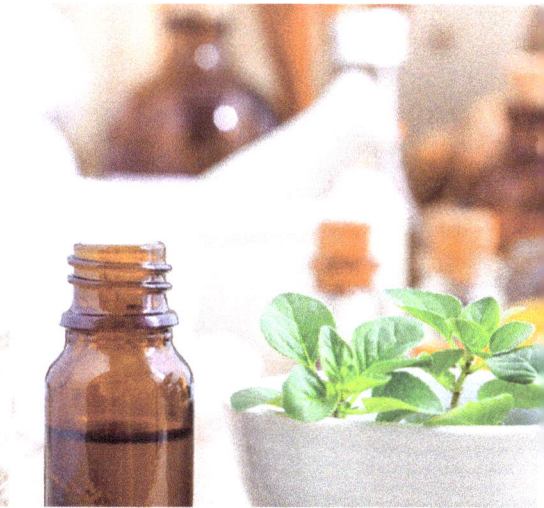

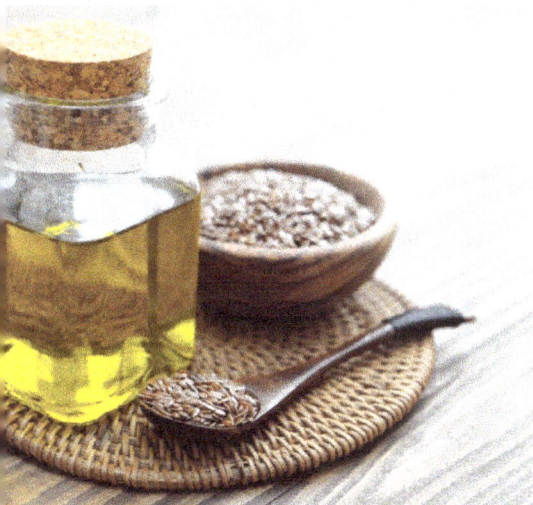

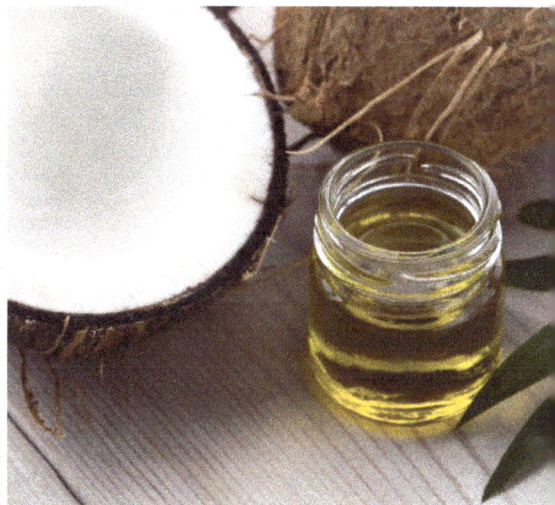

Black seed, oregano, flaxseed and MCT oils provide the body with a great range of good fats and various other micro–nutrients which can serve as a great source of clean energy. They also boost the immune system to help fight off cold or flu more effectively.

Benefits

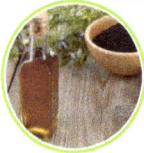

Black Seed oil – has anti–oxidant, anti–inflammatory, anti–viral and anti–fungal properties; may lower blood pressure, blood sugar and cholesterol levels; can help manage allergies; may help reduce symptoms of arthritis; good for skin, hair, brain, heart, bones, respiratory system, reproductive system and digestive system health; can boost the immune system and stimulate production of antibodies due to thymoquinone and other micro–nutrients presence. You may also experience a great sense of well–being and mental clarity after taking this oil.

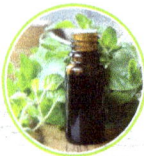

Oregano oil – has anti–oxidant, anti–inflammatory, anti–fungal, anti–viral and anti–bacterial properties; acts as natural antibiotic and pain killer; can help treat yeast infections; may lower cholesterol levels; can help speed up wound healing; may reduce side effects from other medications; good for skin, brain, respiratory system and digestive system health; can boost the immune system due to carvacrol, thymol and other micro–nutrients presence.

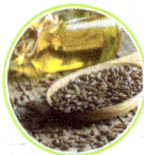

Flaxseed oil – has anti–oxidant and anti–inflammatory properties; high in healthy Omega 3 and Omega 6 fatty acids; can elevate mood and provide energy for body and mind; can reduce blood pressure, cholesterol and blood sugar levels; may help manage arthritis and dry eyes symptoms; can improve menopause symptoms; good for skin, hair, brain, bones, kidneys, digestive system, heart and cardiovascular system health; can boost the immune system due to anti–oxidant and anti–inflammatory properties, omega 3 fatty acids and various other micro–nutrients contents.

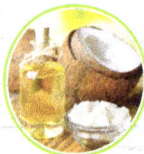

Medium Chain Triglycerides (MCT) – C6, C8, C10 and C12 oils – have anti–bacterial, anti–fungal and anti–inflammatory properties; can elevate mood; can raise metabolism levels; can help balance levels of hormones in the body; help enter the state of ketosis and achieve weight loss goals; may help with diabetes and Alzheimer's disease management; good for hair, nails, brain and digestive system health; can boost the immune system by their natural anti–fungal, anti–viral and anti–bacterial properties and by providing the body and especially the brain with a clean energy source.

Directions

For best well–being and immune system boosting results, it is recommended to take these oils together.

Take 1 teaspoon of black seed oil with 4 drops of oregano oil, followed by one tablespoon of flaxseed oil, followed by one tablespoon of MCT oil. You can dissolve these oils in warm water if you don't like the taste. Most people enjoy taking them straight but everyone is different, so always taste a small amount of each oil and decide for yourself how you prefer to take them. You can also add them to salads or other foods as a dressing.

These oils can be taken once or twice a day—early around 7–8 am upon waking and around 12 pm for the second time. Start with one early morning dose and see how your body reacts before taking these oils more often.

It is also recommended to try these oils separately starting with small doses and gradually increasing the portion sizes.

Where to buy them

You can find the above oils in local retail stores, some pharmacies or online.

Warnings

Don't take the oils described above after 2 pm as they may interfere with sleep quality.

Never overdose on any oils as it may put extra strain on your digestive system which may eventually lead to organ failure.

Read labels carefully to ensure taking correct dosages.

Always seek professional medical advice before adding these oils to your diet if you are pregnant or breastfeeding, to make sure you are not allergic to any of the oils described above and to ensure that you don't have underlying medical health conditions.

WEAPON 19

INCREASE FOOD INTAKE

It is important to increase overall food intake by at least 25% when you are trying to prevent illness or when you are trying to recover from cold or flu.

By consuming more foods than you usually would, you are making sure that your body always has an abundance of the energy, vitamins, macro and micro nutrients necessary for efficient immune system function and speedy recovery.

Make sure that you are eating only nutritious, healthy and natural foods as they possess many immune–boosting health benefits.

Include as many fruits, vegetables, legumes, grains and nuts as possible.

Add extra healthy snacks between meals so your body has sustained energy to fight the illness.

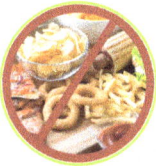

Avoid heavily processed junk foods with artificial flavors, preservatives, bad fats, sugar and various other artificial chemicals as they can be harmful to your health, increase your chances of getting sick and considerably extend your recovery times by making the immune system much weaker.

The next few chapters describe many plant–based foods which should be added to the diet to maximize the chances of avoiding falling ill in the first place and making the recovery process much faster if you are already sick.

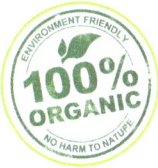

Always try to get all plant–based foods in organic forms if you can – they contain hardly any artificial chemicals and offer health benefits in the most natural form.

Important advice for taking plant-based foods like fruits, vegetables and nuts:

Chew and grind plant–based foods thoroughly for at least 20 seconds before swallowing. Not only will this facilitate digestion, but it will help with sublingual release and absorption of many important vitamins and micro–nutrients that would otherwise be destroyed in the digestive tract.

For best cold and flu–fighting results, take various mixed natural plant–based foods every 3–4 hours in small portions throughout the day.

Warning

Overeating after 6 pm negatively affects sleep quality which weakens the immune system and undermines cold– and flu–fighting efforts.

WEAPON 20

TAKE ORANGES, MANDARINS, TANGERINES AND LEMONS WITH SOME PEEL

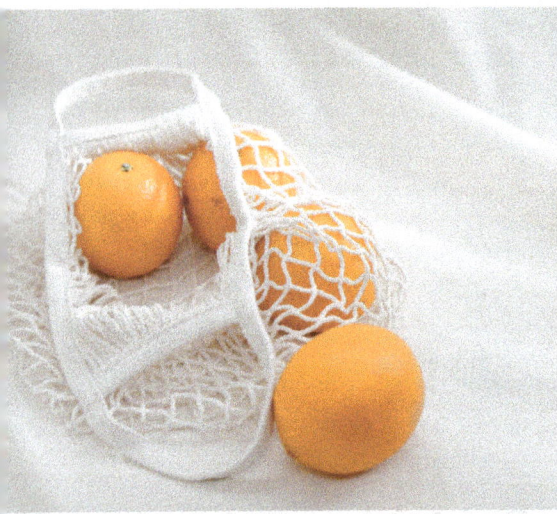

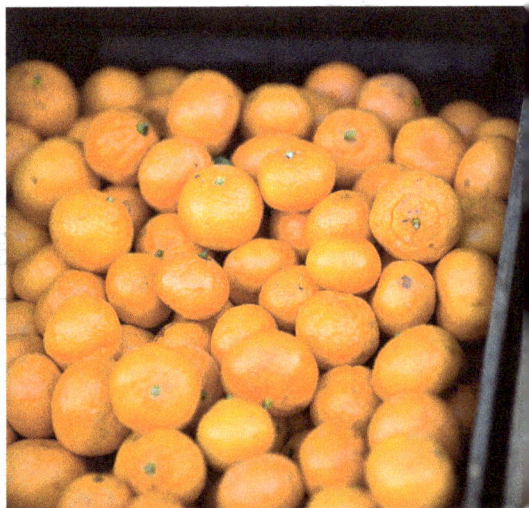

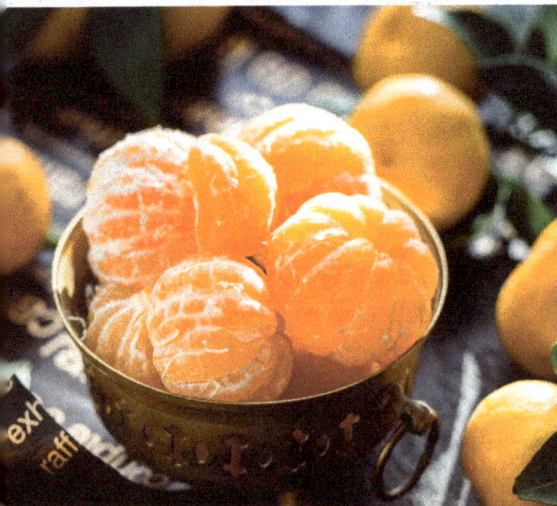

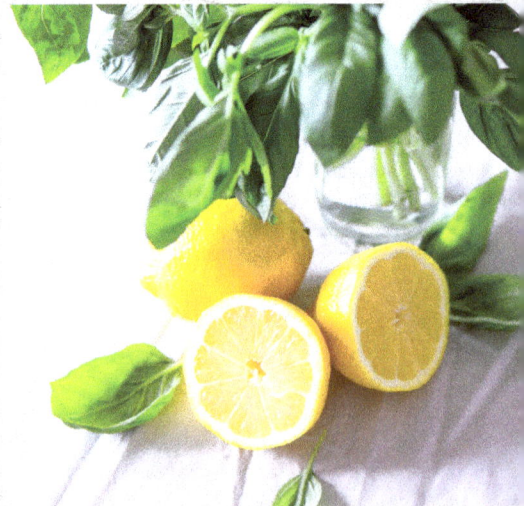

Citrus fruits are a great healthy addition to your diet. Most people are used to eating the inside parts of citrus fruits, but not many would eat the peels. It turns out that citrus fruit peels also provide great benefits to health and contain nutrients that are unique to the peels and are not present in the inside fruit. The next time you eat citrus fruit, think twice before discarding the peels. Keep at least a small part to use as another natural health booster.

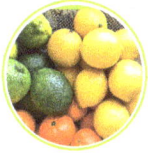

Oranges, lemons, tangerines and mandarins are high in vitamin C, polyphenols, flavonoids and many other important micro–nutrients which enable them to act as potent antioxidants and boost the immune system.

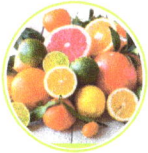

Citrus fruit peels are rich in important micro–nutrients as well and have been used for centuries as remedies for various diseases. They possess anti–fungal and antimicrobial properties which are helpful for the body when fighting off cold or flu.

How to take citrus fruits with their peels

Before eating the inside parts of an orange, mandarin, tangerine or lemon, chew thoroughly a small piece—from about 2 x 2 mm to 1 cm x 1 cm—of organic, fresh and raw (not dried or cooked) orange, mandarin, tangerine or lemon peel. Start by taking very small pieces of the peel and gradually increase the size to about 1 cm x 1 cm portion or a bit larger. Eat the inside part of the citrus fruits after eating a small piece of the peel to soothe the bitter taste.

Take some citrus fruits every 3–4 hours when you are trying to recover from cold or flu. You can alternate oranges, mandarins, tangerines and lemons in the same day or take just the ones you prefer. Mandarin peels usually have milder taste, orange and tangerine peels are somewhere in the middle and lemon peels have the most bitter taste.

You can take lemons with maple syrup, agave nectar or similar sweetener to make their taste more pleasant.

It is best to take citrus fruits in organic form as the peels readily absorb pesticides and other chemicals.

Precaution warning for taking oranges, mandarins, tangerines and lemons with the peels

Citrus fruit peels must only be taken if you have eaten something at least 30 minutes before and must be followed by drinking a warm drink and eating some food because peels may irritate the digestive system and cause heartburn–like symptoms. Stop taking citrus peels if you feel discomfort. Start with very small pieces and gradually increase the size so your digestive system can adapt.

If you are pregnant or breastfeeding, consult a doctor before you start taking citrus fruit peels to ensure you are not allergic to them and that you don't have pre–existing medical conditions that could be aggravated by peels and citrus fruits.

WEAPON 21

EAT A CARROT AND AN APPLE EVERY DAY

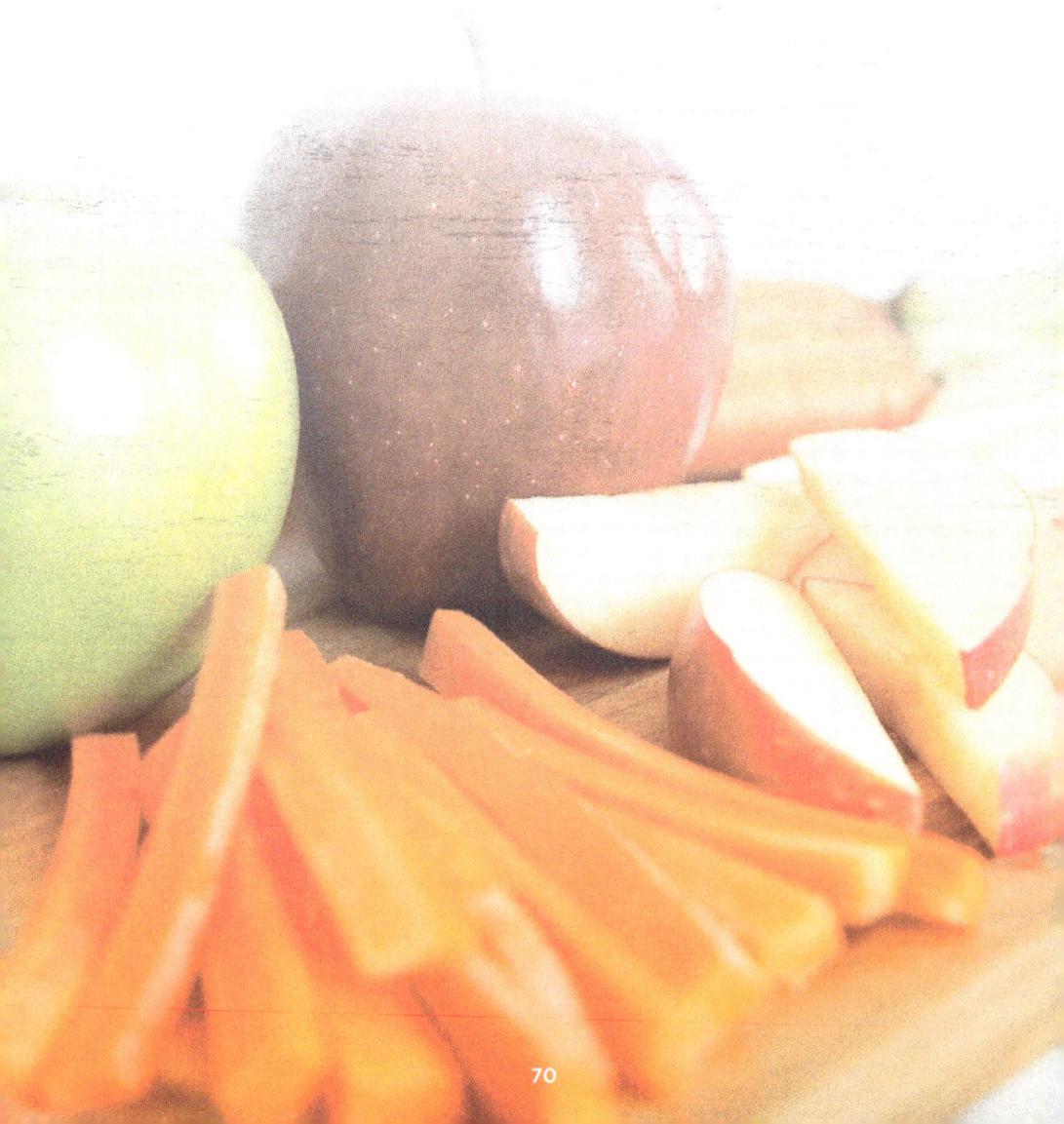

Carrots and apples are rich in vitamins, antioxidants and other important nutrients. They have many health benefits which are multiplied when taken together.

Carrots and apples can help strengthen the immune system, which will increase chances of rapid recovery from cold– or flu–related infections.

People often say that an apple a day keeps the doctors away. This saying should rather be, "a carrot and an apple a day." Together they act as a much stronger natural health and immune system booster.

Some of their benefits include:

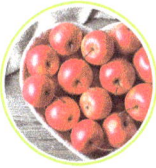

Apples: beneficial for bone, heart, stomach and brain health; can lower risk of diabetes; great for lowering cholesterol levels; have immune boosting properties due to high vitamins, minerals, antioxidants and other micronutrients contents.

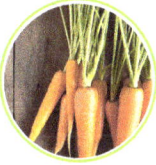

Carrots: good for eye, teeth, skin, hair and liver health; can lower cholesterol and blood pressure levels; very high in vitamins, antioxidants, and other important micronutrients that can help strengthen the immune system.

How to take them

If you like a bit of crunch eat one raw carrot followed by 1 raw apple once or twice a day. If you prefer a milder texture and more flavor, you can grate them and mix together or even place them with some water into a NutriBullet or similar blender for a delicious refresher smoothie. You can also add them to salads.

Take them at midday if you prefer to take them once a day or around 9 am and 2 pm if you are taking them twice.

Don't take them after 3–4 pm as they may affect sleep patterns.

For better health benefits take only organic apples and carrots as their skins can absorb chemicals used in non–organic farming practices.

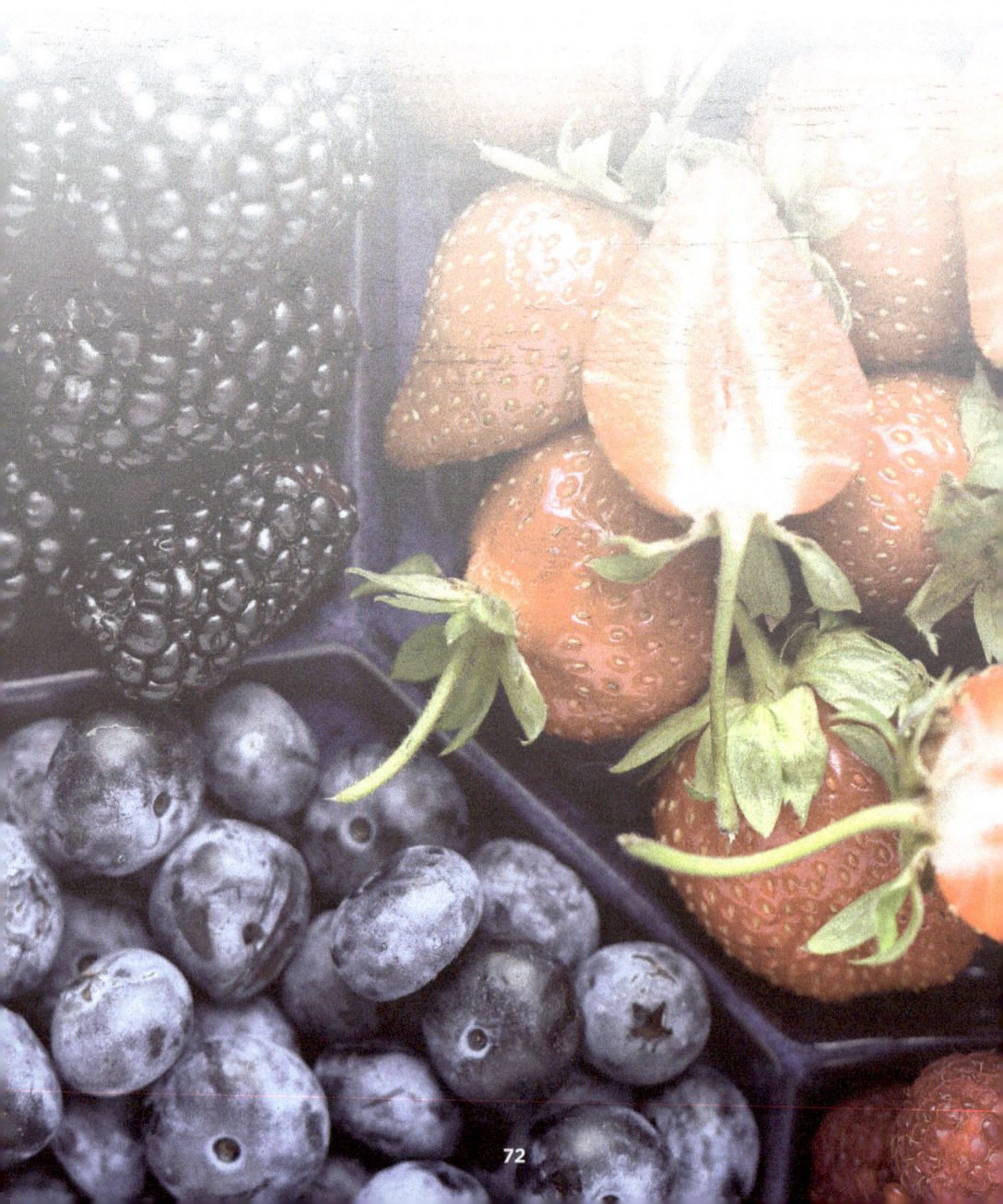

WEAPON 22

BERRIES

Berries are nature's superfoods that can be used effectively when fighting cold or flu. Apart from being a delicious addition to the diet, they possess powerful antioxidant qualities, are packed with important vitamins and minerals that can strengthen the immune system and help us recover from or prevent cold– and flu–related illnesses.

Below are some benefits of eating berries:

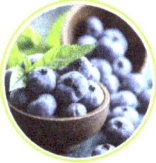

Blueberries – contain anthocyanins, quercetin, kaempferol, myricetin and chlorogenic acid, which are all potent antioxidants; beneficial for healthy skin, bones, heart and digestive system; may lower blood pressure; can improve mental health. Blueberries contain vitamin C and other vitamins, minerals and micronutrients that can strengthen the immune system.

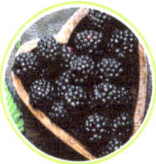

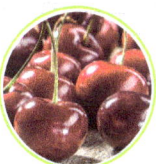

Blackberries – high in antioxidants; good for healthy brain, heart and bones; can assist in weight management; contain vitamin K which improves blood health and circulation; boosts the immune system due to high content of vitamins A, C and other micronutrients.

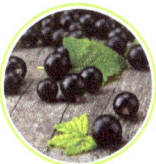

Blackcurrants – high in antioxidants; can reduce inflammation in the body; good for skin, heart, eyes, brain, liver and kidneys health; may lower blood pressure and cholesterol levels; can improve digestion; high in vitamin C and other vitamins, minerals and micronutrients which can boost the immune system.

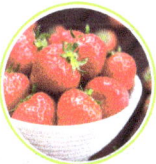

Strawberries – high in antioxidants; have anti–inflammatory properties; beneficial for eye, skin, brain and heart health; can reduce cholesterol and regulate blood pressure levels; high in vitamin C, other vitamins, minerals and micronutrients that together can help boost the immune system.

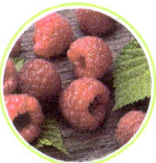

Raspberries – high in antioxidants; good for skin, heart, bones and brain health; can improve digestion; have anti–inflammatory action; may prevent diabetes; high in vitamin C and other vitamins, minerals and micronutrients that can strengthen the immune system.

Cherries – tart or sweet variety – high in antioxidants; possess anti–inflammatory properties; beneficial for heart and hair health; contain melatonin which can improve sleep; can lower blood pressure due to potassium content; may improve cardiovascular and digestive health; can lower cholesterol level; may help with arthritis; contain high amounts of vitamin C and polyphenols which can boost the immune system.

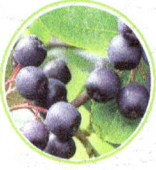

Acai berries – Acai berries have been used as a medicine for decades and are considered a superfood worldwide for good reason. Some benefits of taking Acai berries include: very high in antioxidants; beneficial for heart, skin and brain health; possess anti–aging properties; promote healthy digestion; can reduce cholesterol level; can boost the immune system due to high anthocyanins, vitamins, minerals, various other micronutrients contents and by stimulating the production of gamma delta T cells and white blood cells interleukin 12 (IL–12) along with myeloid cells which are necessary for healthy immune system function.

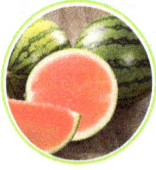

Watermelon – yes it is a berry, although a very big one and with big health benefits: contains powerful antioxidants lycopene and vitamin C which have anti–inflammatory properties; beneficial for eyes, bones, skin, hair, gums digestive system and heart health; great for staying hydrated; can prevent heat strokes; can lower blood pressure; boosts the immune system due to high antioxidant lycopene, vitamins C, B6 and vitamin A contents.

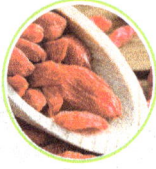

Goji Berries – high in antioxidants; have anti–inflammatory properties; good for skin, liver and eyes health; can lower blood sugar and cholesterol levels; may increase testosterone levels; can boost the immune system due to high vitamins A, C, minerals and various micronutrients contents.

How to take them

For most health benefits, take all of the above listed berries in organic form. Non–organic berries can contain high amounts of chemicals that can harm your health.

Mix approximately 100 to 200 grams of each berry listed above in a big air–tight container and keep them in your freezer. Consume at least 50 grams of mixed berries every 3 hours while you are sick to ensure that you are constantly receiving the vitamins, minerals and micronutrients necessary to boost the immune system.

Take acai berry in organic freeze dried or organic frozen pulp forms, unless you can get fresh acai at a local health store or online. Ensure it is 100% acai berry product without additives.

Take Goji berries in dried or frozen organic form.

If you can't find all the berries listed above, try to get at least few of them and take them mixed together. This way you will get diverse antioxidants, vitamins, minerals and many other micronutrients beneficial for the immune system.

Don't eat berries after 5 pm as they may interfere with sleep. The only berries recommended before sleep are cherries. They contain melatonin which can help you sleep better.

WEAPON 23

EAT MORE FRUIT

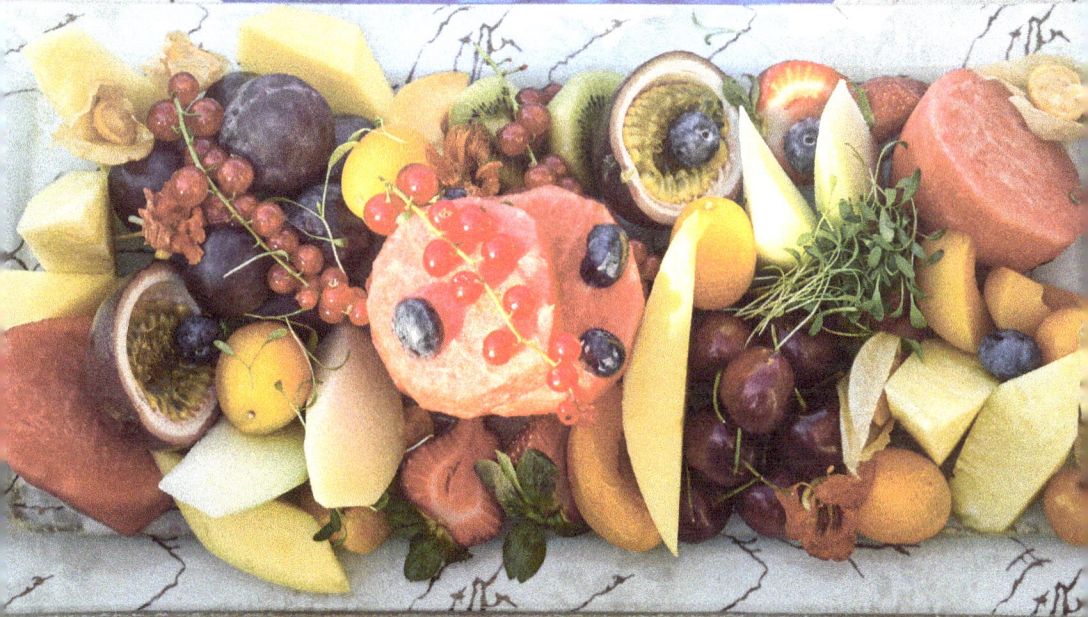

Most fruits are very healthy natural foods packed with various antioxidants, vitamins, minerals and other beneficial nutrients that work together to support the weakened immune systems when we are getting sick and not feeling our best.

Below are some benefits of adding fruit to the diet when you are fighting cold or flu

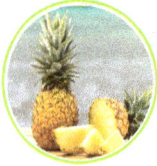

Pineapples – have anti–oxidant and anti–inflammatory properties; can help with weight loss; can help prevent and treat respiratory illnesses due to vitamin C and bromelain; may relieve arthritis and prevent asthma; may reduce blood clotting; can relieve nausea; may improve sleep; can lower blood pressure and improve blood circulation; can strengthen gums; good for eyes, hair, skin, bones, heart and digestive system health; can boost the immune system due to high vitamin C and other vitamins, minerals and other micronutrients contents.

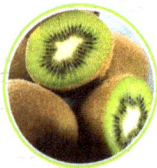

Kiwi fruits – have anti–oxidant and anti–inflammatory properties; can lower blood pressure; can help treat asthma; may protect and prevent DNA damage; can improve sleep quality; may help manage blood pressure and reduce blood clotting; good for eyes, skin, lungs, bones, heart and digestive system health; contain vitamin C, anti–oxidants and other vitamins, minerals and micronutrients that can boost the immune system.

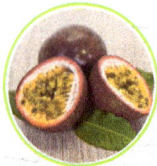

Passionfruits – have anti–oxidant and anti–inflammatory properties; may help with diabetes and improve insulin sensitivity; can improve sleep quality and calm nerves; may lower blood pressure and improve circulation; may assist with staying healthy during pregnancy; may improve respiratory tract ailments; good for eyes, skin, bones, brain, digestive system and heart health; can boost the immune system due to vitamin C, vitamin A and other vitamins, minerals and micronutrients contents.

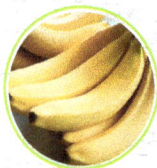

Bananas – have anti–oxidant and anti–inflammatory properties; contain amino acid tryptophan, which can help improve memory and mood; may reduce menstrual pain; can improve sleep; can help with anaemia; may lower blood pressure and blood sugar levels; can relieve stomach ulcers; beneficial during pregnancy; good for skin, eyes, kidneys, digestive system and heart health; can boost the immune system due to vitamin C and other vitamins, minerals and micronutrients contents.

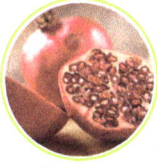

Pomegranates – have anti–oxidant and anti–inflammatory properties; can fight off fungal and bacterial infections; can improve memory; can act as blood thinner; may reduce stress levels; may improve erectile dysfunction; can lower dental plaque formation; may prevent Alzheimer's disease and arthritis; may reduce blood sugar levels and insulin resistance; can lower blood pressure; good for skin, hair, bones, brain, heart and digestive system health; can boost the immune system due to vitamin C and other vitamins, minerals and micronutrients contents.

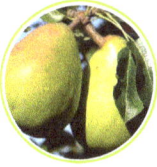

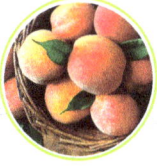

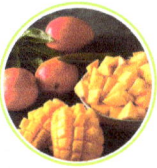

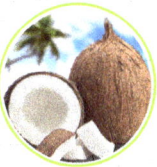

Pears – have anti–oxidant and anti–inflammatory properties; may lower blood pressure; may lower chances of getting type 2 diabetes; good for hair, skin, bones, cardiovascular, heart and digestive system health; can boost the immune system due to vitamin C and other vitamins, minerals and micronutrients contents.

Peaches – have anti–oxidant and anti–inflammatory properties; beneficial during pregnancy; may help with lowering allergy symptoms; may lower blood pressure; may help calm the mind; good for skin, eyes, brain, bones, heart and digestive system health; can boost the immune system due to vitamin C and other vitamins, minerals and micronutrients contents.

Mangoes – have anti–oxidant and anti–inflammatory properties; beneficial during pregnancy; can lower cholesterol levels; may help prevent diabetes; have aphrodisiac effect; good for eyes, skin, hair, brain, heart and digestive system health; can boost the immune system due to vitamin C and other vitamins, minerals and micronutrients contents.

Coconuts – yes it sound like a nut, but it's usually classified as a fruit – most people who are allergic to nuts can safely eat coconuts with no adverse reactions (but it's still good to check with your doctor in case you are allergic before adding them to your diet) – have anti–oxidant, anti–inflammatory, anti–fungal, anti–viral and anti–bacterial properties; have high amounts of MCTs which provide the body and especially the brain with a great clean source of energy; can help with staying hydrated; may help with blood sugar control; good for teeth, skin, brain, thyroid, kidneys, bladder, digestive system and heart health; can boost the immune system due to MCTs, manganese and other vitamins, minerals and micro–nutrients contents.

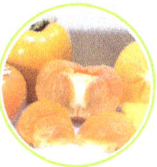

Persimmons – have anti–oxidant and anti–inflammatory properties; may regulate blood sugar and lower cholesterol levels; good for eyes, skin, brain, bones, liver, digestive system and heart health; can boost the immune system due to vitamin C, vitamin A and other vitamins, minerals and micro–nutrients contents.

Apart from the benefits listed above fruits are also a great source of fibre and are relatively low GI foods that will make you feel "full" longer and will help with weight loss as a result. Most fruits can also help with detoxification of the body.

How to take them

As with berries, take some mixed fruits every 3–4 hours when you are sick or as a preventive measure.

Don't eat fruits after 5 pm as they may interfere with sleep. The only fruits that are safe to take before bed are bananas, passion fruits and kiwi fruits. To improve sleep quality, take 1 banana, 1 kiwi and 1 passionfruit about 2–4 hours before going to sleep.

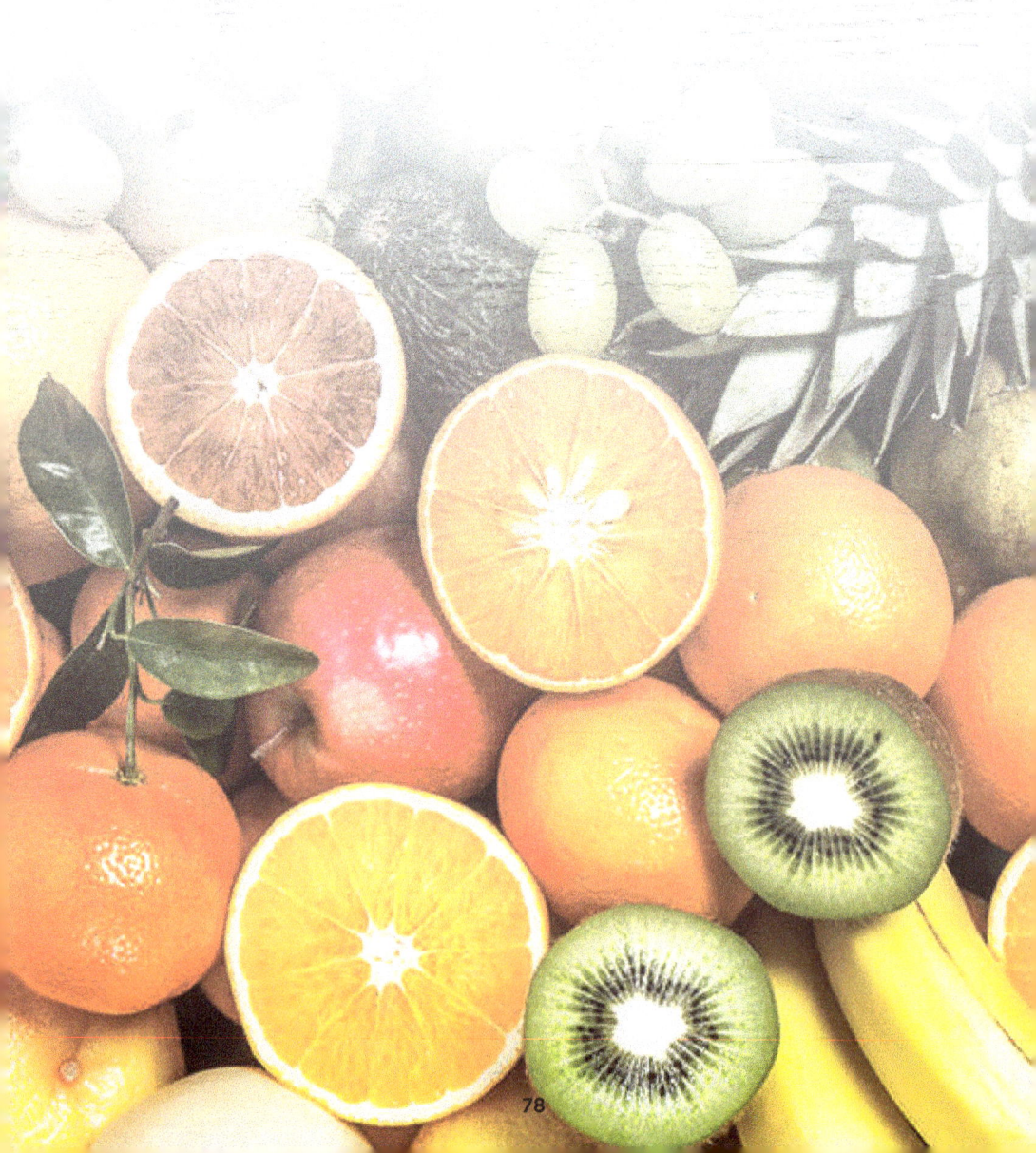

WEAPON 24

VEGETABLES AND GREENS

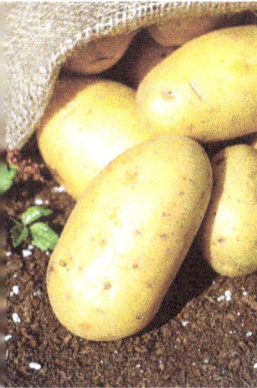

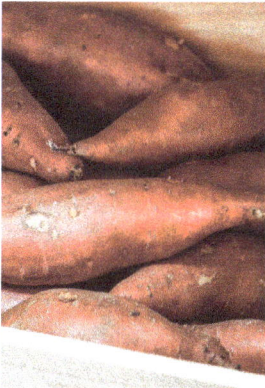

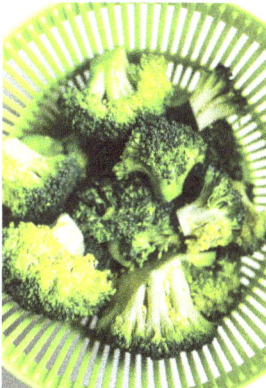

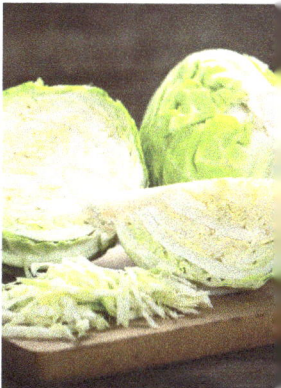

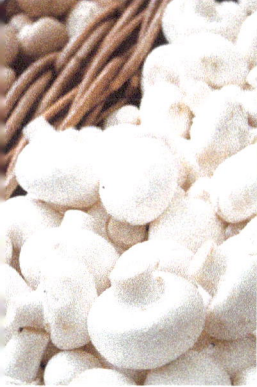

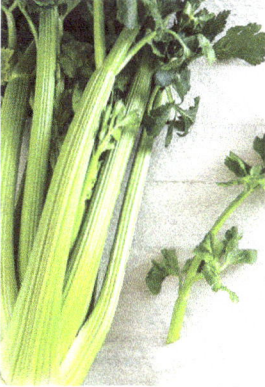

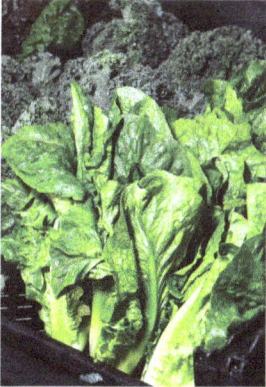

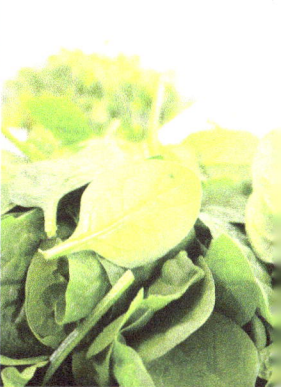

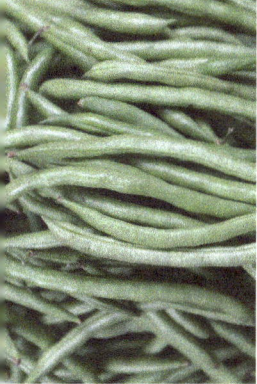

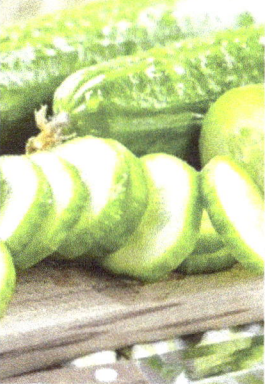

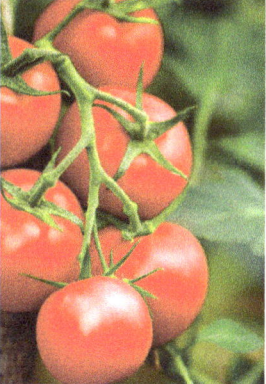

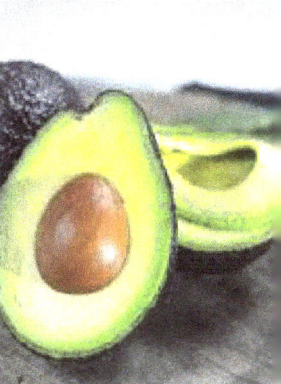

Vegetables and greens are great sources of carbohydrates, protein, fiber, vitamins, minerals, antioxidants and many other indispensable nutrients that the body and immune system require to stay healthy, energized and effectively fight cold– and flu–related diseases.

Always make sure that you consume a healthy mix of vegetables and greens described in this chapter when you are trying to prevent getting sick or when you are already sick and trying to recover as soon as possible.

Described below are some of the benefits of taking vegetables and greens

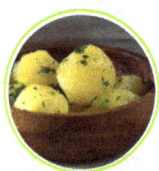

Potatoes (boiled, steamed or baked – not fried) – have antioxidant and anti–inflammatory properties; can regulate blood pressure and decrease acidity in digestive tract; good for skin, bones, brain, heart and digestive system health; contain resistant starch which is beneficial for gut bacteria and blood sugar control; can boost the immune system due to high vitamin C, vitamins B and various other minerals and micronutrients contents.

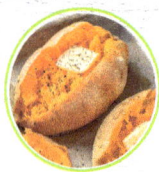

Sweet Potatoes (boiled, steamed or baked – not fried) – have anti–inflammatory and anti–microbial properties; can improve fertility and lower blood pressure; beneficial for eyes, hair, skin, cardiovascular system, brain and gut health; can boost the immune system due to high vitamins A, C and various other vitamins, minerals and micronutrients contents.

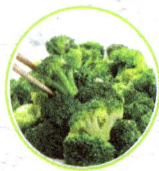

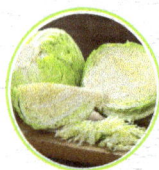

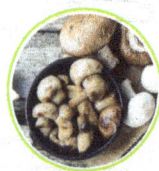

Broccoli (steamed, stir fried or boiled) – anti–oxidant and anti–inflammatory properties; good for digestive system, heart, brain, joints, bones, eyes and skin health; can lower blood sugar and cholesterol levels; boosts the immune system due to high vitamin C and various other vitamins, minerals and micronutrients contents.

Cabbage (white or red – steamed or boiled) – anti–oxidant and anti–inflammatory properties; can lower blood pressure and cholesterol levels; can offer protection against radiation; can be used as a hangover cure; can treat ulcers; beneficial for heart, skin, brain and digestive system health; can boost the immune system due to high vitamin C and various other vitamins, minerals and micronutrients contents.

White Button Mushrooms (raw, boiled or stir fried) – potent anti–oxidant and anti–inflammatory properties; good for bones, brain and heart health; may help prevent diabetes; can lower cholesterol levels; contain vitamin D and polysaccharides which can boost the immune system.

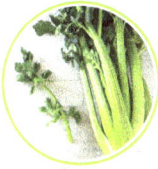

Celery (raw) – contains more than twelve potent antioxidants; can lower inflammation in the body; can stimulate neurogenesis, beneficial for brain, digestive and cardiovascular system health; can lower blood pressure and cholesterol levels; boosts the immune system due to high vitamin C and various other vitamins, minerals and micronutrients contents.

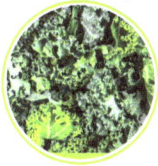

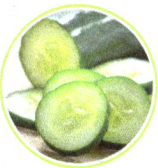

Kale (raw) – possesses potent antioxidant and anti–inflammatory properties; lowers cholesterol; good for eyes, skin, hair, heart, liver, digestive tract and bones health; contains high amounts vitamin C and various other vitamins, minerals and micronutrients which can boost the immune system.

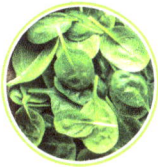

Spinach (raw) – acts as an antioxidant; has anti–inflammatory properties; can help manage diabetes and blood sugar levels; good for heart, eyes, skin, hair, bones and digestive system health; can lower blood pressure; can boost the immune system due to high vitamin C, vitamin A and various other vitamins, minerals and micronutrients contents.

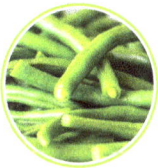

Green Beans (raw, steamed or stir fried) – anti–oxidant and anti–inflammatory properties; lower cholesterol and blood pressure levels; good for nails, skin, hair, bones, eyes and heart health; beneficial during pregnancy; high in iron which can help with anaemia; may detoxify the body; can boost the immune system due to vitamin A, vitamin C and various other vitamins, minerals and micronutrients contents.

Cucumbers (raw) – have anti–oxidant and anti–inflammatory properties; help keep your body hydrated; may lower blood pressure and blood sugar levels; can prevent diabetes; good for brain, eyes, hair, skin, bones, digestive system, heart and cardiovascular system health; may detoxify the body; can boost the immune system due to various anti–oxidants, vitamins, minerals and other micronutrients contents.

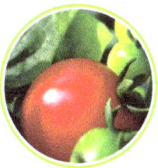

Tomatoes (raw) – contain potent antioxidant lycopene and other antioxidants which together offer many health benefits; have anti–inflammatory properties; may lower blood sugar levels; can help restore damage done by smoking; may help with blood clotting and wound healing; may prevent kidney stones; good for hair, skin, eyes, bones, digestive system, cardiovascular and heart health; can boost the immune system due to vitamin C and various other vitamins, minerals and micronutrients contents.

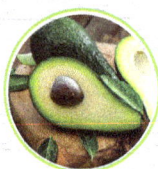

Avocados (raw) – technically avocados are berries, but they are mostly classified as vegetables due to common use – have potent anti–oxidant and anti–inflammatory properties; can lower cholesterol and triglycerides levels; beneficial during pregnancy; may help relieve enlarged prostate symptoms; help detoxify the body; may help with managing arthritis; may help absorb plant–based nutrients and anti–oxidants; can boost fertility; may prevent Alzheimer's and Parkinson's neurodegenerative diseases; may help lose weight; have anti–microbial properties; good for eyes, skin, brain, bones, digestive system and heart health, can boost the immune system due to vitamin C and other vitamins, minerals and micronutrients contents.

How to take vegetables and greens

Eat some mixed vegetables and greens described above every 3–5 hours when you are trying to recover from cold or flu. For best results mix as many vegetables and greens as you can and take them together. Take cooked, boiled or stir–fried vegetables separately from raw ones – you can mix all raw vegetables as a salad and eat them first followed by the mix of cooked ones. You can use a little soy sauce, salt, vinegar or other desired seasoning. Don't overdose on salt as it may lead to harmful health consequences.

Immune Boosting Power Salad

Slice 1 medium tomato, 1 medium cucumber, 1 stick of celery, about 50 grams of kale and mix together. Then add 50 grams of raw spinach leaves, 50 grams of sprouted mung beans (or any other sprouts), 1 to 2 tablespoons of pine nuts, 1 to 2 tablespoons of raisins, 1 tablespoon of nutritional yeast (optional), 1 tablespoon of apple cider vinegar and a little salt. Give it another good stir and the salad is ready.

Eat this salad at least once a day around midday. It can also be taken 2 times a day, in the morning and at lunch time.

This salad will make you feel full of energy and will elevate your mood. It will also provide the body with many necessary nutrients like vitamins, minerals and antioxidants that will help fight off cold or flu.

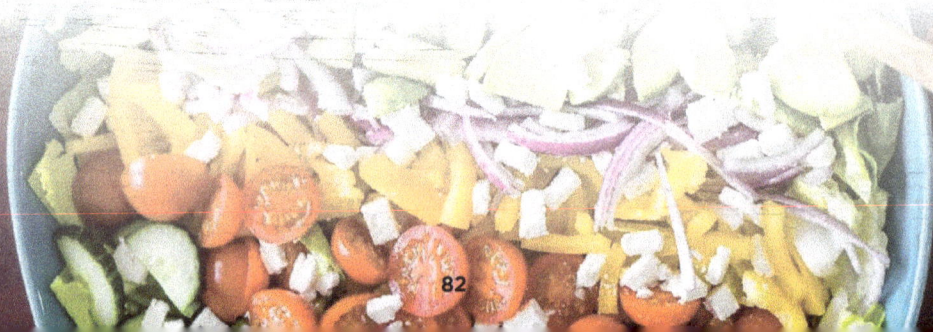

WEAPON 25

LEGUMES, GRAINS AND SEEDS

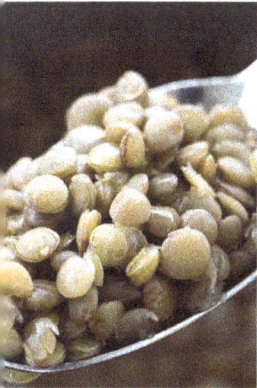

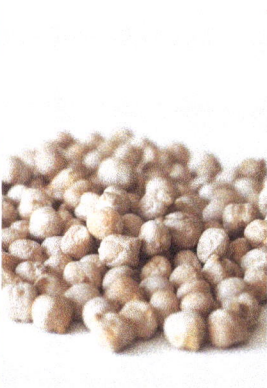

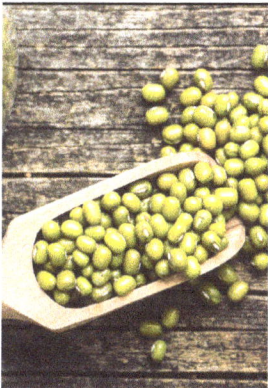

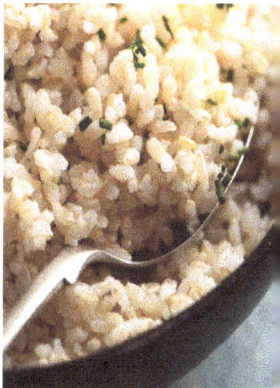

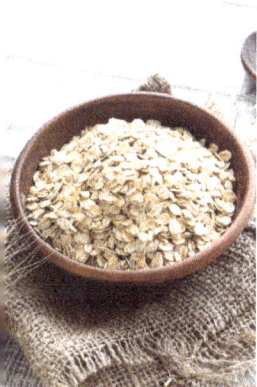

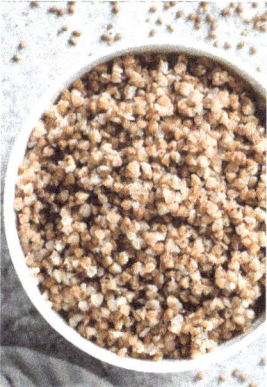

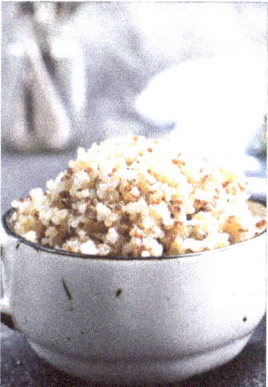

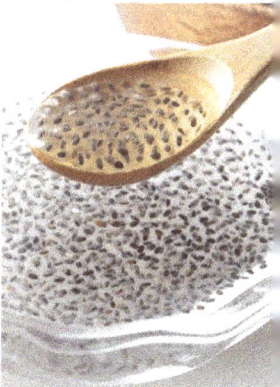

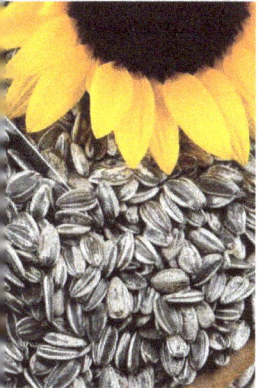

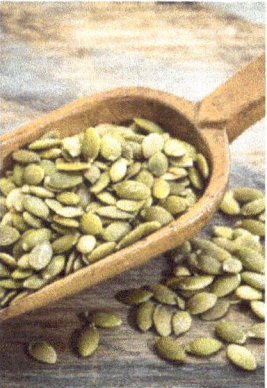

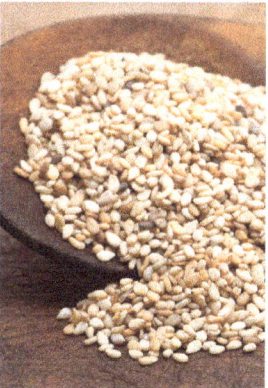

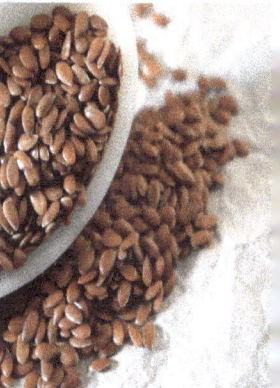

Legumes, grains and seeds are a great addition to the cold– and flu–fighting arsenal. They are a good source of protein, fiber, healthy fats and carbohydrates along with many vitamins, minerals, anti–oxidants and micronutrients that provide us with sustained energy levels and help strengthen the immune system, which is important when fighting off cold– or flu–related infections.

Always consume plenty of varied legumes, grains and seeds when you are avoiding getting sick or when you are fighting existing cold or flu.

Below are some benefits of taking legumes, grains and seeds

Legumes

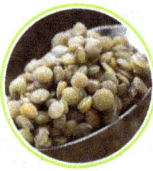

Lentils (cooked or steamed) – have potent anti–oxidant properties due to high polyphenols contents; can lower cholesterol and stabilize blood sugar levels; beneficial during pregnancy; good source of plant–based iron; high in protein; good for nails, skin, hair, bones, heart and digestive system health; can boost the immune system due to high protein and various other vitamins, minerals and micronutrients contents.

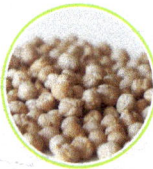

Chickpeas (Garbanzo beans—cooked or steamed) – have anti–oxidant and anti–inflammatory properties; high in protein; can help prevent or manage diabetes by controlling blood sugar levels; beneficial during pregnancy; contain iron and can prevent anaemia; may lower cholesterol and blood pressure levels; good for hair, eyes, skin, brain, bones, colon, cardiovascular system, heart and digestive system health; can support the immune system due to high protein and various other vitamins, minerals and micronutrients contents.

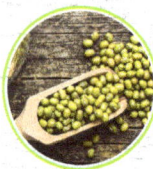

Mungbeans (cooked or steamed) – have anti–oxidant, anti–inflammatory, anti–fungal and anti–microbial properties; high in protein; may lower cholesterol, blood pressure and blood sugar levels; beneficial during pregnancy; may prevent heat stroke; good for skin, hair, cardiovascular system, heart and digestive system health; can boost the immune system due to high protein and various other vitamins, minerals and micronutrients contents.

Grains

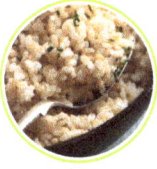

Brown rice (cooked or steamed) – gluten free; antioxidant and anti–inflammatory properties; may lower cholesterol levels; may reduce the risk of getting type 2 diabetes and gallstones; good for bones, nervous system, cardiovascular system, heart and digestive system health; can boost the immune system due to selenium and various other vitamins, minerals and micronutrients contents.

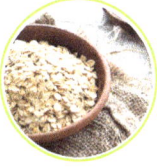

Oats (cooked or steamed) – anti–oxidant and anti–inflammatory properties; may prevent childhood asthma; can lower blood pressure, blood sugar and cholesterol levels; can improve sleep; can prevent constipation; good for skin, cardiovascular system, heart, colon and digestive system health; can boost the immune system due to beta–glucans and various other vitamins, minerals and micronutrients contents.

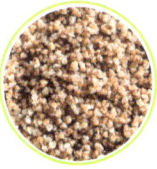

Buckwheats (cooked or steamed) – it is actually a seed but mostly referred to as a grain – gluten free; have anti–oxidant and anti–inflammatory properties; can reduce blood sugar levels and help manage diabetes; can lower cholesterol and blood pressure; can help prevent gallstones; source of complete plant–based protein; good for skin, heart and digestive system health; can boost the immune system due to various vitamins, minerals and other micronutrients contents.

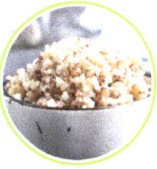

Quinoa (keen–wah cooked or steamed) – technically a seed but commonly referred to and used as a grain – gluten free; anti–oxidant and anti–inflammatory properties; good source of complete plant based protein; very high in fiber; contains unique flavonoids quercetin and kaempferol; can help treat anaemia; can reduce blood sugar and cholesterol levels; beneficial during pregnancy; good for hair, skin, bones, cardiovascular system, heart and digestive system health; can boost the immune system due to high protein, various vitamins, minerals and micronutrients contents.

Seeds

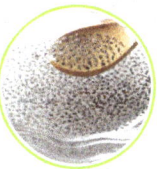

Chia seeds (soaked in water) – anti–oxidant and anti–inflammatory properties; very high in fiber; good source of plant–based protein and omega–3 fatty acids; can lower cholesterol and blood pressure levels; can convert fast carbohydrates into slow ones; may help with managing diabetes and blood sugar levels; good for skin, bones, brain, cardiovascular system, heart and digestive system health; can boost the immune system due to high protein, omega 3s, various vitamins, minerals and micronutrients contents.

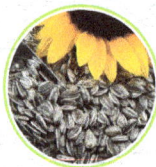

Sunflower seeds – have anti–oxidant and anti–inflammatory properties; good source of healthy fats and protein; can lower blood pressure, cholesterol and blood sugar levels; beneficial during pregnancy; may help detoxify the body; can elevate your mood; good for hair, skin, nervous system, bones, cardiovascular system, heart and digestive system health; can boost the immune system due to protein, selenium, zinc, various vitamins, minerals and micronutrients contents.

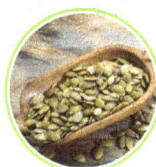

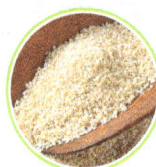

Pumpkin seeds (pepitas) – anti–oxidant and anti–inflammatory properties; good source of protein and plant–based omega 3 fatty acids; beneficial during pregnancy; can lift your mood; contain magnesium, zinc and tryptophan, which can improve sleep; may reduce cholesterol and blood pressure levels; can lower blood sugar levels and help prevent or control type 2 diabetes; good for hair, bones, heart, reproductive system (especially in men), liver, prostate and bladder health; can boost the immune system due to protein, zinc, various vitamins, minerals and micronutrients contents.

Sesame seeds – anti–oxidant and anti–inflammatory properties; contain iron which can improve and prevent anaemia; may lower cholesterol, blood pressure and blood sugar levels; may help with arthritis; may improve mood; good for skin, teeth, hair, thyroid, bones, lungs, respiratory system, digestive system and heart health; can boost the immune system due to protein, zinc, selenium, various vitamins, minerals and other micronutrients contents.

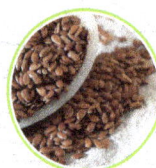

Flaxseeds – have anti–oxidant and anti–inflammatory properties; great source of plant–based protein, lignans and omega–3 fatty acids; may reduce hot flashes and arthritic pain; may lower cholesterol, blood pressure and blood sugar levels; good for skin, cardiovascular system, heart and digestive system health; can boost the immune system due to protein, omega–3s, various vitamins, minerals and micronutrients contents.

How to take legumes, grains and seeds

Take some mixed legumes, grains and seeds every 3–4 hours through the day when you are fighting off cold or flu. For best results and to get a complete plant–based protein amino acids profile, always take legumes mixed with some grains and seeds preferably in equal proportions. You can take them a few hours apart separately in bigger portions as well, but make sure that in the same day you consume equal amounts of each substance so that you get enough of the necessary amino acids from their plant–based proteins.

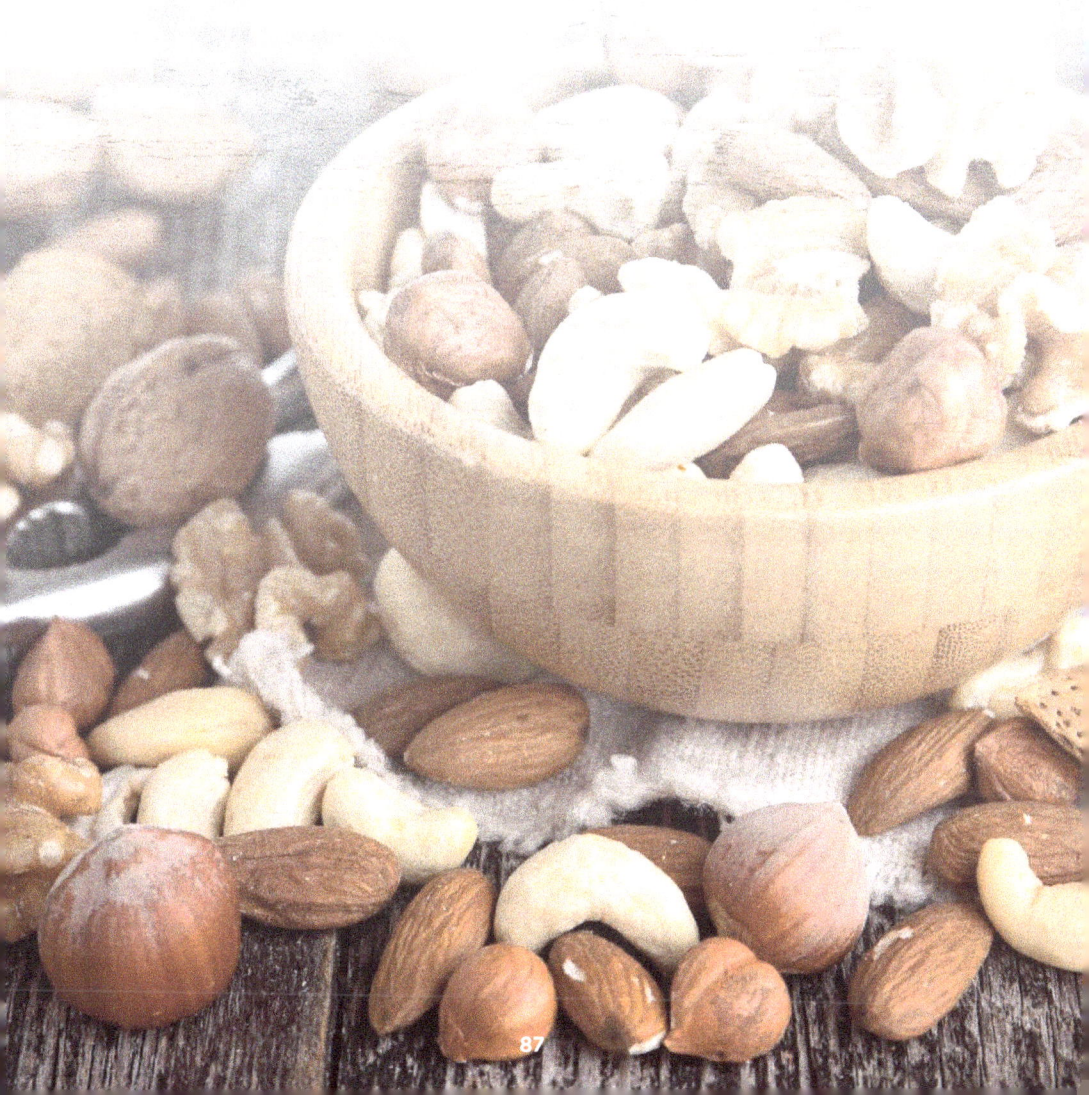

WEAPON 26

EAT NUTS

Nuts pack a real punch when it comes to strengthening the immune system and fighting cold– or flu–related diseases. They are full of healthy fats, good quality proteins, a variety of vitamins, anti–oxidants, minerals and various other micronutrients which have great potential to help prevent or recover from cold and flu.

Always include a mixed variety of nuts in your diet when you are trying to recover from cold– or flu–related infections.

Some health benefits of taking nuts

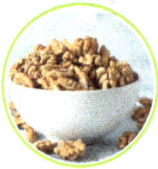

Walnuts – anti–oxidant and anti–inflammatory properties; great source of protein and omega 3 fatty acids; can elevate mood; may lower blood pressure, blood sugar and cholesterol levels; can improve sleep quality; beneficial during pregnancy; good for skin, hair, nails, bones, brain, heart, nervous system, cardiovascular system, reproductive system (especially in men) and digestive system health; can boost the immune system due to protein, healthy fats, various vitamins, minerals and micronutrients contents.

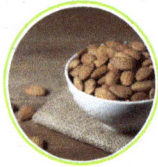

Almonds – anti–oxidant and anti–inflammatory properties; may lower blood pressure, blood sugar and cholesterol levels; may prevent and help treat type 2 diabetes; high in vitamin E; beneficial during pregnancy; good for skin, hair, brain, teeth, bones, digestive system, heart and cardiovascular system health; can boost the immune system due to high vitamin E, healthy fats, protein, various vitamins, minerals and other micronutrients contents.

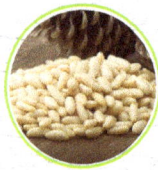

Pine Nuts – anti–oxidant and anti–inflammatory properties; may lower blood sugar levels and help control type 2 diabetes; may lower cholesterol levels; can elevate mood; beneficial during pregnancy; good for eyes, skin, hair, brain, heart, cardiovascular system and digestive system health; can boost the immune system due to vitamin E, zinc, protein, healthy fats, various other vitamins, minerals and other micronutrients contents.

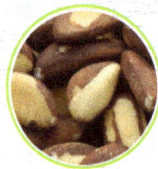

Brazil Nuts – anti–oxidant and anti–inflammatory properties; high in selenium; can improve your mood; can lower cholesterol, blood sugar levels and help with type 2 diabetes; may increase testosterone levels; good source of healthy fats and protein; good for skin, bones, brain, heart, digestive system and thyroid health; can boost the immune system due to high selenium, protein, healthy fats, vitamins, minerals and other micronutrients contents.

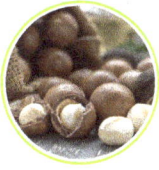

Macadamia Nuts – anti–oxidant and anti–inflammatory properties; may lower blood sugar levels and help with type 2 diabetes management; may lower blood pressure and cholesterol levels; good for skin, hair, teeth, bones, brain, heart, nervous system, digestive system and cardiovascular system health; can boost the immune system due to protein, healthy fats, various vitamins, minerals and other micronutrients contents.

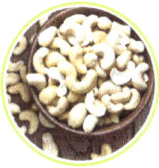

Cashew Nuts – anti–oxidant and anti–inflammatory properties; may elevate mood and increase relaxation; good source of protein and healthy fats; can lower cholesterol levels; may lower blood sugar levels and help control type 2 diabetes; can reduce blood pressure; may prevent gallstones; may help with anaemia due to iron presence; good for eyes, skin, hair, teeth, brain, bones, heart, nervous system, blood, cardiovascular system and digestive system health; can boost the immune system due to protein, healthy fats, copper and various other vitamins, minerals and micronutrients contents.

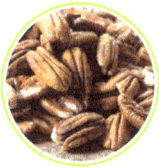

Pecan Nuts – anti–oxidant and anti–inflammatory properties; good source of protein and healthy fats; may lower cholesterol levels; can lower blood sugar levels and help with type 2 diabetes management; good for hair, skin, nervous system, brain, bones, heart and cardiovascular system health; can boost the immune system due to high magnesium, protein, healthy fats, zinc, manganese, vitamin E and various other vitamins, minerals and micronutrients contents.

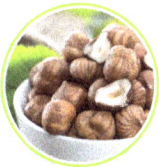

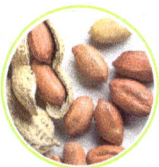

Hazelnuts – anti–inflammatory and anti–oxidant properties; good source of protein; contain omega–3 and omega–6 healthy fats; can elevate mood; beneficial during pregnancy; may lower blood pressure and cholesterol levels; can lower blood sugar and help prevent and manage type 2 diabetes; good for skin, hair, heart, cardiovascular system, brain, nervous system, bones, joints, prostate, reproductive system and digestive system health; can boost the immune system due to protein, healthy fats, vitamin E and various other vitamins, minerals and micronutrients contents.

Peanuts – technically they are legumes but mostly used and perceived as nuts – anti–oxidant and anti–inflammatory properties; good source of healthy fats and protein; may prevent gallstones; may lower blood sugar and cholesterol levels; good for hair, skin, brain, cardiovascular system, heart and digestive system health; can boost the immune system due to protein, healthy fats, copper, vitamin E and various other vitamins, minerals and micronutrients contents.

How to take them

Mix about 100 grams of each above–described nuts in a small container and take 1–2 pieces of each nut every 3–4 hours throughout the day as a preventive measure while you are at risk or when you are sick and recovering from cold or flu.

If you can't find all of the nuts listed above, try to at least find walnuts, almonds, pine nuts and brazil nuts as they provide the most health benefits of the nuts listed above.

For better nutrients profile and to facilitate digestion, it is highly recommended to soak the nuts in cold or slightly warm water for at least 3 to 8 hours before taking them. They will taste much better and have much softer texture.

Warnings about nuts

Double check with your doctor that you are not allergic to nuts before taking them. Many people are allergic to some nuts, especially to peanuts.

All nuts are very high calorie foods, so they should be consumed in moderation to avoid weight gain and sleep problems.

Don't eat too many nuts after 3 pm as they are high in calories and will keep you awake at night.

The only nuts that can be safely taken before sleep are walnuts and almonds – they can help your sleep. Don't take more than one whole walnut and 3–5 almonds as overeating will keep you awake.

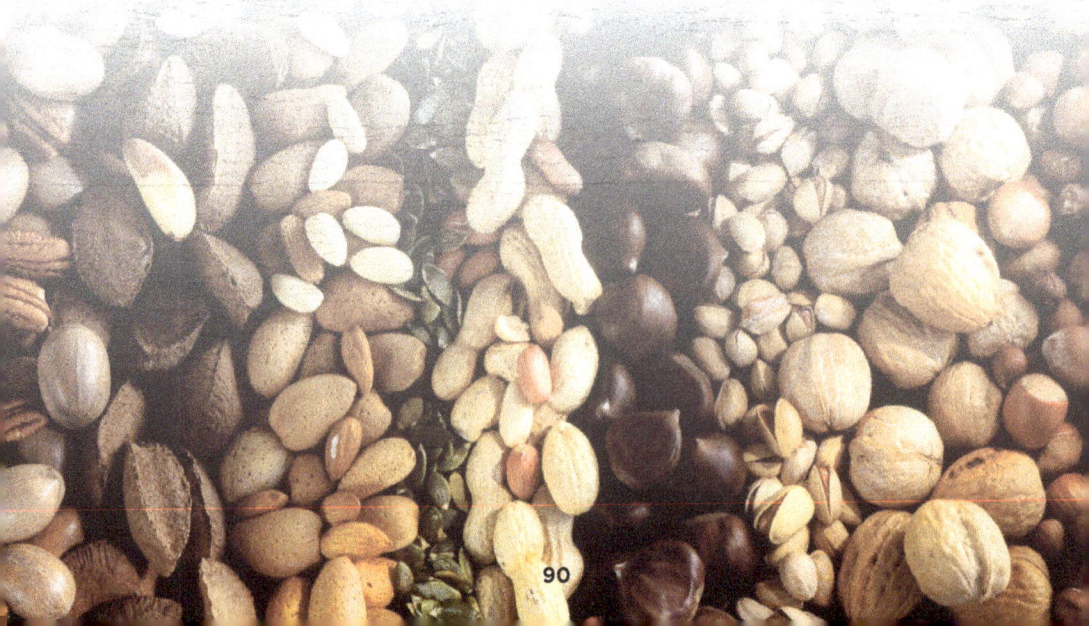

AVOID ANIMAL–BASED AND HIGHLY PROCESSED FOODS HIGH IN SUGAR, BAD FATS AND GLUTEN

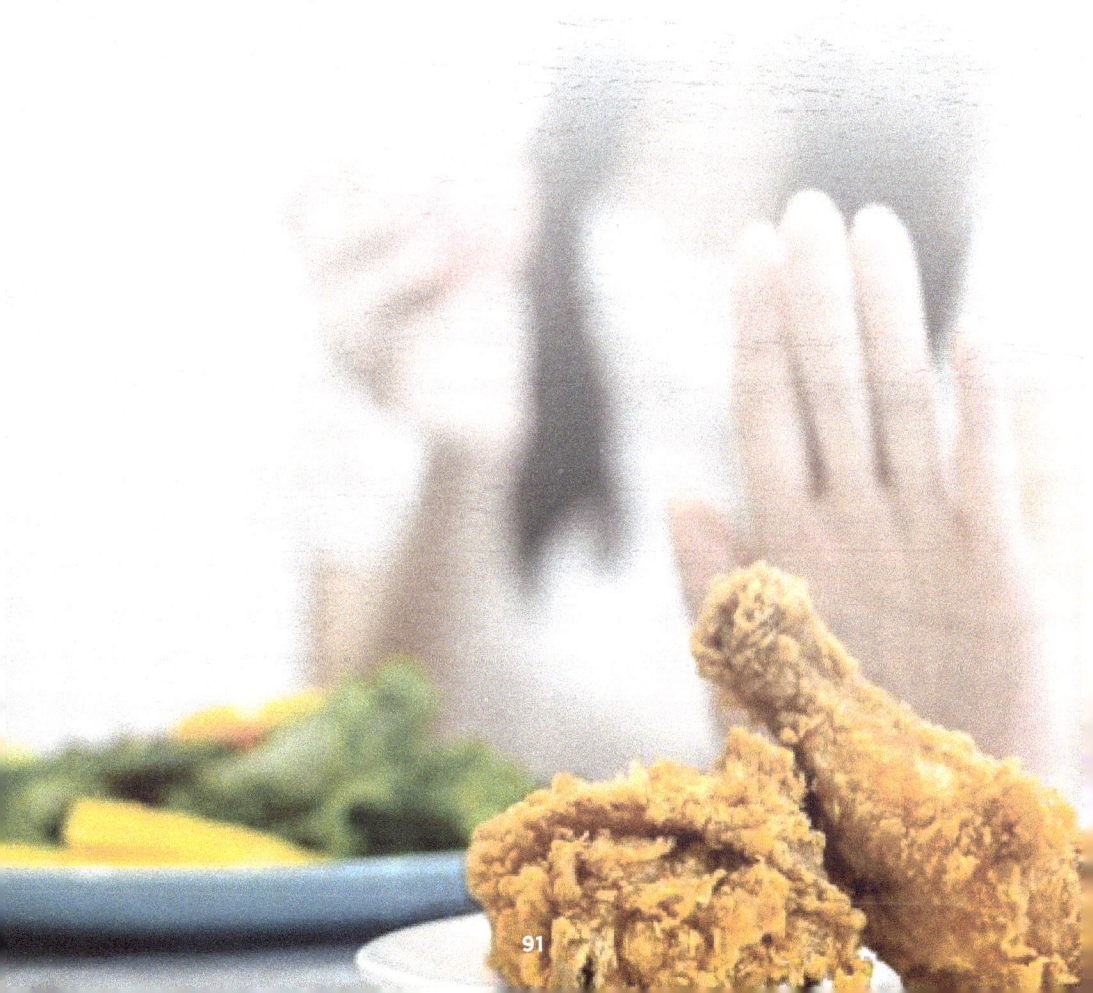

Animal–based and highly processed foods can worsen illness and weaken the immune system. Such foods often increase chances of getting sick and significantly increase cold and flu recovery times.

Listed below are some negative health effects of harmful foods that you should avoid:

Bad fats

Don't eat too much fatty foods. Especially avoid saturated fats and foods that contain trans fats. All fatty foods that solidify at rooms temperature contain some saturated fats – saturated fats can increase blood cholesterol levels, which may be harmful to your health. Foods that contain saturated fats – most meats and animal products; dairy products – milk, cream, cheese and whey protein; coconut oil, palm oil and cocoa butter.

Trans fats are most harmful to your health and must be completely avoided especially when you are trying to recover from cold or flu. Trans fats can increase the levels of bad cholesterol and inflammation in the body and can decrease the levels of good cholesterol which may lead to higher risk of cardiovascular diseases and weaker immune system response. Foods that contain trans fats – most fried and processed foods contain some amount of trans fats. Read labels carefully to make sure there are no trans fats in the foods you intend to consume.

Refined sugars

Limit consumption to whole foods like fruits and some sweet vegetables that contain naturally occurring sugars in combination with fiber and other nutrients. Avoid drinking too much fruit juices on their own as they spike your blood sugar levels much more than if taken with other foods. Try your best to avoid foods that have added white sugar or fructose as they will lead to increase in blood sugar levels – this especially applies to sugary soft drinks as they contain a lot of refined sugars.

Avoid taking refined sugars and fructose on their own at all costs as they lead to negative health effects like weaker immune system; increased blood pressure and cholesterol levels; problems with teeth and gums; faster aging; may increase stress levels; weight gain; increase your risk of getting diabetes, Alzheimer's, cardiovascular and various other diseases.

Avoiding refined sugars will also lead to many health benefits like – better looking skin; improved digestion; gradual healthy weight loss; continuous and stable energy levels throughout the day without sudden crashes when you need to resort to coffee or another sugary drink to keep going; better overall mental performance, feeling of well–being and healthier body; improved sleep quality; healthier and stronger immune system.

Gluten

It is highly recommended to minimize or avoid gluten–containing foods, especially when recovering from or preventing cold or flu.

Gluten has many potential negative effects on health even for people who don't have celiac disease – you may feel tired and experience brain fog symptoms after consuming it; it may cause digestive system discomfort; some people may experience skin problems similar to eczema, dermatitis and psoriasis; it may cause inflammation in the gut and trigger an immune system response; may damage gut microbiome, which can lead to problems digesting various foods; may increase the risk of getting various auto–immune diseases; may increase intestinal permeability which may lead to unwanted particles entering your bloodstream.

Some benefits of eliminating gluten from your diet include – increased and more stable energy levels and clearer mind throughout the day; better digestion and no digestive system discomfort after eating; improved athletic performance; better immune system response.

Ensure that you take adequate amounts of fiber–rich foods when you eliminate gluten from your diet.

White rice and processed foods that contain white flour

These foods are very high in refined simple carbohydrates that can spike your blood sugar levels which can lead to unstable energy levels throughout the day and make you experience "crashes" or low energy periods. Always opt for lower GI complex carbohydrate natural foods which don't cause blood sugar surges and contain higher levels of fiber and a variety of other beneficial micronutrients, vitamins and minerals. Choose brown rice and wholemeal flour–based breads and baked goods.

Some benefits of replacing white rice and white flour–based products with brown rice and wholemeal flour–based foods – you will avoid overeating and feel "full" for longer as these foods digest at a slower rate and provide gradual and longer lasting energy release; reduced acidity and inflammation levels in the body; improved digestive system health and healthier gut microbiome; lower risk of heart disease, type 2 diabetes and metabolic syndrome; staying fit and avoiding unwanted weight gain; improved mental performance and improved immune system function.

Animal products - meats, seafood and dairy

Apart from great environmental and ethical reasons, avoiding animal products also offers many health benefits.

Regular consumption of processed and unprocessed meats, seafood and dairy products increases the chances of getting Alzheimer's, cardiovascular and heart diseases, diabetes and stroke. Fats found in most animal products are mostly saturated and can lead to high cholesterol levels and higher risk of cardiovascular diseases.

All meats, especially seafood products, start to decompose the moment the fish or animal dies, so by the time the meat or seafood products end up on the dinner plate they are already full of harmful microbes and bacteria. To reduce spread of bacteria and microbes in most commercially available seafoods and meats, manufacturers add various harmful chemicals and preservatives to delay the decay process, which can lead to even more harmful consequences for overall health.

Some benefits of avoiding animal products include – younger looking body and skin; improved athletic performance; higher and more stable energy levels throughout the day; better brain function; lower cholesterol and blood pressure levels; avoiding unwanted weight gain; healthier heart and digestive system; improved immune system function.

It has been proven by various scientists that avoiding animal products can help reverse heart disease, arthritis and various chronic diseases.

Most animal products require a great deal of energy to digest and contain harmful chemicals, bacteria and microbes, which on their own can cause defensive immune system response, which in turn can lead to weaker immune system and higher risk of getting cold– or flu–related diseases.

To better understand the benefits of avoiding animal–based products, I highly recommend the documentaries Game Changers and Forks over Knives.

Avoiding bad fats, animal products, gluten and high sugar highly processed foods will ensure that the immune system functions properly and at its maximum capacity which will maximize chances of rapid faster recovery from cold, flu and various other diseases.

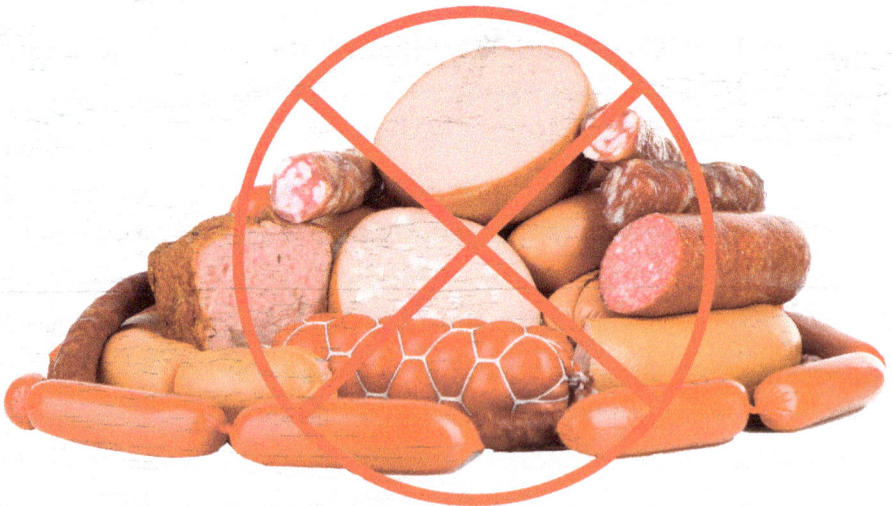

WEAPON 28

REST AS MUCH AS POSSIBLE AND GET ADEQUATE SLEEP

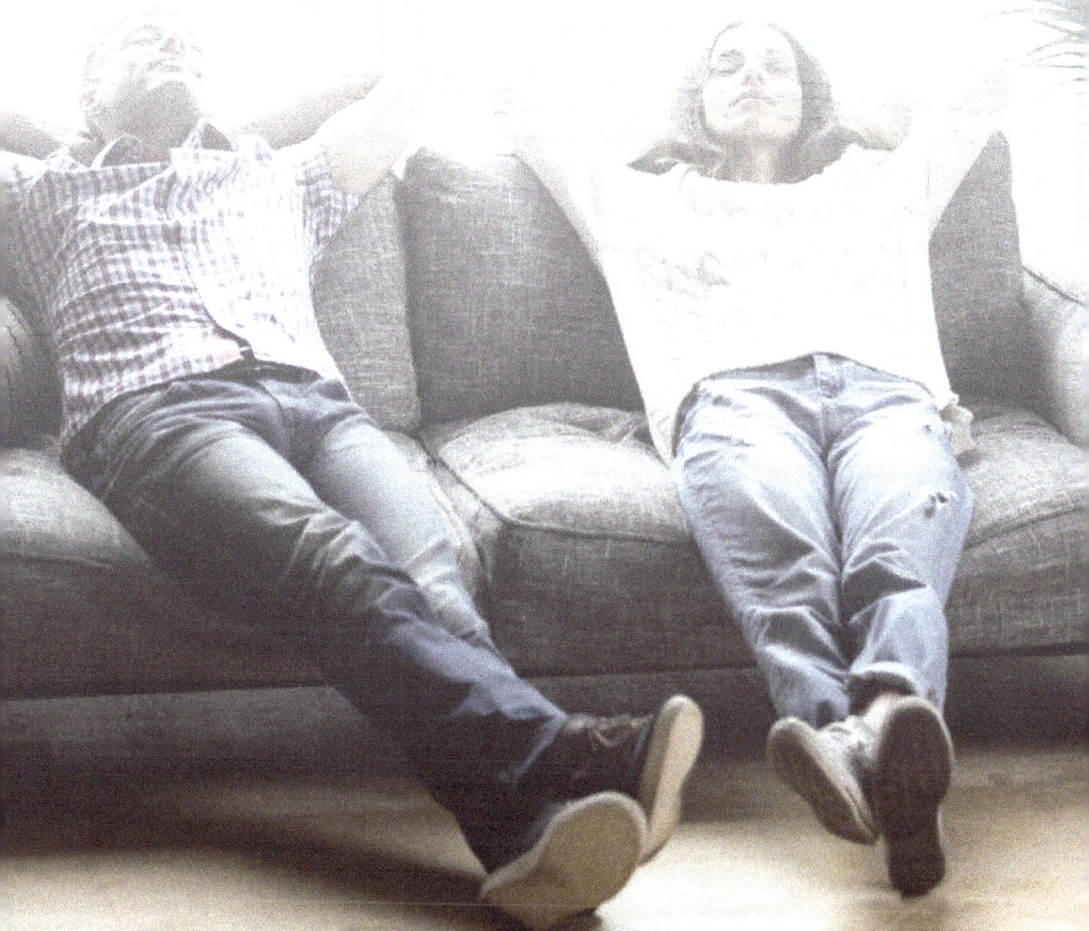

Sleep deprivation and fatigue can rob us of energy, make us feel tired and eventually lead to a weaker immune system response. All these factors make it easier to get sick with cold or flu–related diseases and significantly increase recovery times.

Always get adequate rest when fighting off cold or flu–related illness. Try to lie down for about 10–30 minutes at least twice during the day. You can lie with eyes closed or even sit and rest while reading a book, listening to music or watching a movie. Don't overload your body and brain; save necessary energy to fight the disease.

If possible, taking an 11 am 15–minute power nap is highly recommended. Just set an alarm to exactly 15 minutes when you lie down. This power nap will make you feel refreshed, improve energy levels and a feeling of well–being. It will also boost the immune system which will make your cold or flu recovery times much shorter. Don't take this power nap after 12 pm as it may interfere with sleep patterns and make it hard to fall asleep and stay asleep at night. Avoid making this power nap longer than 15 minutes so you don't go into a deep state of sleep. Doing so will make it difficult to get up. You will feel tired and groggy if you nap longer than 15 minutes.

Another important aspect is to consistently get adequate sleep – go to bed early and sleep at least 7–8 hours. Go to bed and get up at the same time every day, so your body develops regular sleeping patterns. For the best and most refreshing night's sleep, aim to get to bed no later than 10 pm or even before and wake up at 6–7 am so you have time and energy the next day. Dim the lights around you at least 3 hours before you go to sleep and don't use electronic devices with bright screens before bed as bright light and focused mental efforts can make you feel wakeful and disrupt normal serotonin production. Don't eat heavy meals and drink too much water or other drinks after 6 pm. Avoid smoking, drinking caffeine and alcohol containing beverages. Don't eat foods that contain too much refined sugars or too much fat – and don't overeat after 6 pm. Some of the best foods to eat before bed time are: oatmeal with sour cherries, 2–3 halves of walnuts, kiwis, passion fruits and bananas.

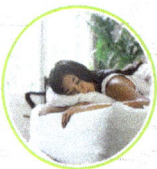

Sleep boosting after–dinner mini meal – This sleep–boosting mini meal can significantly improve sleep quality. Place 3 heaped tablespoons of organic instant oats, about 5–10 frozen or fresh sour cherries and 2–3 crushed halves of walnuts into a bowl and pour about half a glass of boiling water over the oat mixture. Wait for about 10–15 minutes until the oats absorb the water and become soft and then enjoy your meal. After this eat one fresh, medium–sized kiwi, 1 passion fruit and follow up with one ripe medium–sized banana. You can also add the frozen pulp of the passion fruit to the oatmeal to save time. This mini meal will give you a mix of good fiber, carbs, protein and fats and other necessary micronutrients to keep you sleeping throughout the night. Take this mini–meal not later than 7:30 pm to ensure that your digestive system is not "busy" while you sleep.

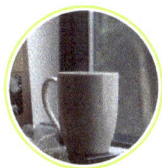

Magic Sleep Tea – For even better quality of sleep, you can try my favorite "Magic Sleep Tea." Place half a teaspoon of dried chamomile, quarter to half teaspoon of dried valerian root, one heaped teaspoon of blended rice and pea vegan protein powder mix, a pinch (approx. 500 mg to 1 gram) of vitamin C powder (ascorbic acid) and a half to one teaspoon of raspberry jam in a cup and fill 30% of the cup with boiling hot water. Mix everything well with a spoon and let it steep for about 5 minutes. Don't pour more than 30% of hot water into the cup as drinking too much before bed could make you wakeful. Drink this "Magic Sleep Tea" approximately 15 to 30 minutes before going to bed. It will improve the quality of your sleep and make you feel more refreshed the next morning.

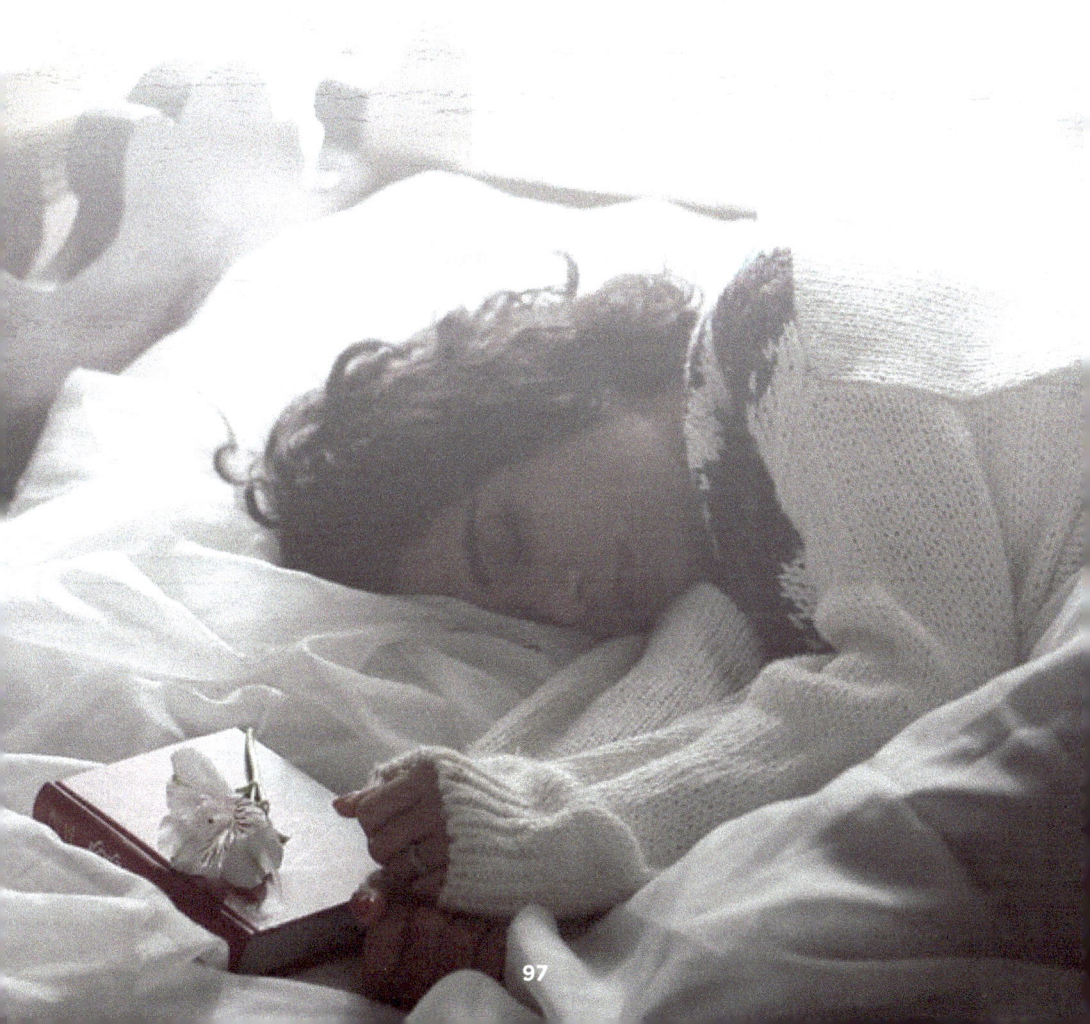

WEAPON 29

STAY WARM. MAINTAIN
GOOD PERSONAL HYGIENE.
KEEP YOUR BODY MOVING
AND EXERCISE REGULARLY.
AVOID CONTACT WITH
PEOPLE SHOWING COLD OR
FLU SYMPTOMS.

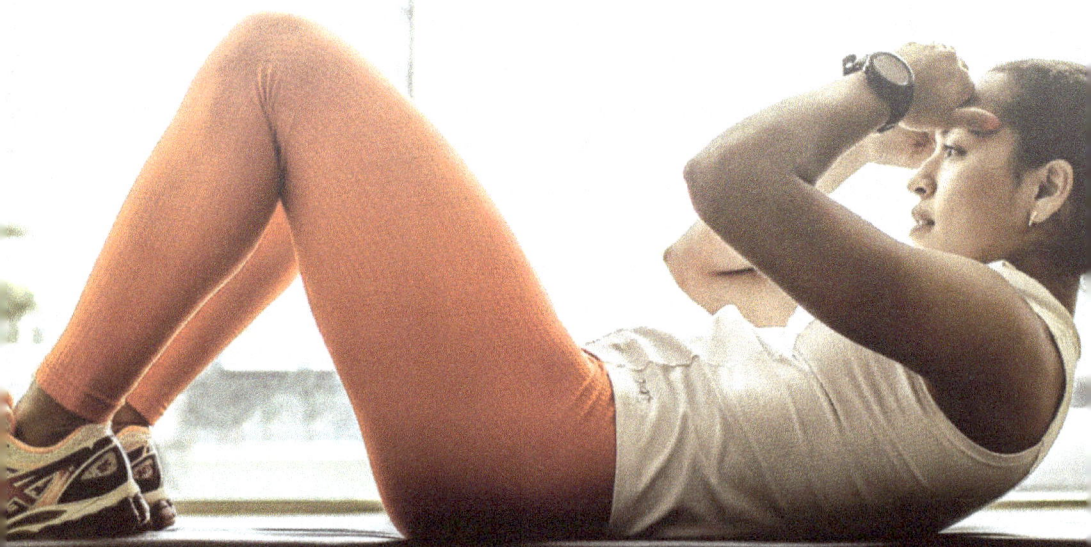

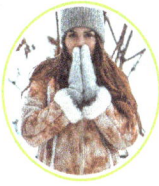

Keep your body warm at all times!
Getting your body cold is one of the main causes of cold and flu. Always keep your body warm – especially feet, hands, chest, neck and head. Use a heater in your home so you stay warm and comfortable. Wear warm clothes in cold weather conditions, avoid drinking cold drinks, eating ice cream or other cold or frozen foods and avoid exposure to cold winds and breezes. Often you may get cold after eating ice–cream, drinking cold beverages or getting exposed to cold weather, cold breezes and winds.

Keep your feet, neck and throat warm! Always! Wear a scarf, double– or triple–warm socks and warm shoes in cold and windy weather.

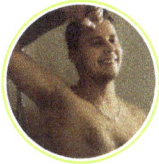

Take prolonged hot showers and baths
Don't get chilled after you take a hot shower or bath. Dry yourself and quickly don warm clothes appropriate to the current weather conditions.

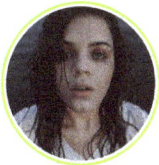

Avoid going out with wet hair or in wet clothes
In cold weather or in a windy conditions. This can weaken the immune system and increase chances of "catching" cold or flu.

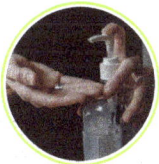

Maintain good personal hygiene
Wash your hands regularly and maintain good hygiene. Take warm showers and wash your clothes and linen regularly. Wash your hands after going out and visiting public places. Brush your teeth at least twice a day, first thing in the morning and just before going to sleep.

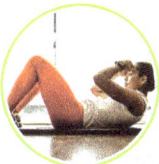

Keep your body moving and exercise regularly
Make sure to follow a very light and regular exercise program at least 2–3 times a week even while you are a little sick. Regular exercising is a proven way to boost the immune system. At least go for short walks to keep you active. Moving your body mobilizes the lymph which carries white blood cells and ensures that the immune function is at its peak state.

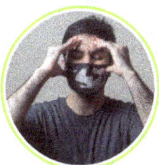

Avoid close contact with people who appear to have symptoms of cold or flu
Avoiding contact with people who have cold or flu is a proven way to prevent yourself from falling sick. This step can prevent airborne or person–to–person transmissions of cold or flu–related infections.

FINAL THOUGHTS AND RECOMMENDATIONS

This book contains many proven methods which can help you avoid sickness or quickly fight off cold– and flu–related illness.

I highly recommend trying all the "Weapons" described in this book. Test them one by one and see how they work for you. Every person is unique, so what works for others may work for you in a different way or not work at all.

Eventually, continue using only the effective "Weapons," the ones which work for your body. Use them any time you feel that you are at risk or when you start experiencing the first symptoms of cold or flu.

It shall be repeated again that one of the most important things when you are trying to prevent or recover from disease is to have a positive attitude and believe beyond any trace of a doubt that you will not get sick in the first place or recover very quickly if you do. You must just know it as if you have already recovered. And of course apart from this belief and knowledge, you have to take active and determined action as early as possible at the first signs of symptoms and every hour of every day even if you think you are at risk or when you already have symptoms. This way you will recover much faster or not get sick at all.

It took more than ten years for me to find the natural and effective cold and flu fighting "weapons" presented in this book. I had to find them one by one through trial and error. The best advice I got from doctors when I was sick was to take Panadol and antibiotics which did not help me much and sometimes made me feel even worse.

I sincerely wish you – the reader of this book – to find weapons that effectively work for you and which will help you recover from cold– and flu–related diseases much faster or prevent you from getting sick altogether.

Everyone deserves to always feel good, but cold and flu can deprive us of the valuable and limited productive time resources that we have in this life. This will not be the case for you if you know how to actively and effectively fight these illnesses using the right methods and strategies.

Thank you for reading this book and may you always be healthy, vibrantly youthful, strong and happy!

September 2020
Halekulani, NSW Australia